EARLY SIRENS

CRITICAL HEALTH WARNINGS & HOLISTIC MOUTH SOLUTIONS
FOR SNORING, TEETH GRINDING, JAW CLICKING,
CHRONIC PAIN, FATIGUE, AND MORE

DR. FELIX LIAO, DDS

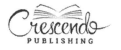

Crescendo
PUBLISHING

Early Sirens
by Dr. Felix Liao, DDS

Cover Design By Melody Hunter
Copyright © 2017 by Dr. Felix Liao

ISBN: 978-1-944177-91-1 (P)
ISBN: 978-1-944177-92-8 (P-Color)
ISBN: 978-1-944177-93-5 (E)

Crescendo Publishing, LLC
300 Carlsbad Village Drive
Ste. 108A, #443
Carlsbad, California 92008-2999
1-877-575-8814

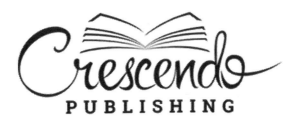

A Note from the Author

Sleep apnea is on the rise, along with stress, healthcare cost, and your copay and your health insurance premium. What can you do to reduce your health risks while looking better and feeling great? How can you head off sleep apnea and its many costly complications proactively?

In *Six-Foot Tiger Three Foot Cage (6T3C)*, we focused largely on establishing the sleep-airway-mouth link. This sequel builds on that link to offer a model of proactive care for the human frame.

Many clues are scattered on health's downhill slide toward sleep apnea and its medical-dental-mental-financial consequences. Putting on Sherlock Holmes' hat to do some Chair Side Investigation™ (CSI) leads all too often to an impaired mouth structure as the culprit. An Impaired Mouth starts your health domino toward sleep apnea and its co-morbidities. *Early Sirens* shows you the dots to connect, and what you can do.

Sleep apnea is simply a late outcome of Impaired Mouth Syndrome, a diverse set of medical, dental, mental symptoms stemming from the discrepancy between a size 3 mouth and a size 6 tongue resulting in a partially choked airway.

Sleep apnea happens because the critical health warnings from the body have not been heard early on. This causes patients to waste massive amounts of time and energy going from doctor to doctor to seek answers and resolutions they're not finding — until now. What clues are on the earlier part of the downhill, and how can the slide be slowed or even reversed?

Early Sirens follows the "WholeHealth paradigm" that says all parts of the body are connected without the artificial/academic medical-dental-mental divides. *Early Sirens* then offers a proactive program called Holistic Mouth Solutions™ that redevelops your "size 3 jaws" to open your airway, support your sleep, and realigning your jaws with head and spine reduces or resolves chronic pain naturally.

In short, restoring your health starts with restructuring your mouth following the law of better form and function. This is the missing piece in the sleep apnea puzzle.

At the end of each chapter, I offer a few Holistic Mouth Nuggets – "take-away pearls" on the WholeHealth perspective. Holistic Mouth Nuggets are simply conclusions that have made sense to me and worked for my patients. They have not been validated by formal studies. Until all the studies are in, "Does this make common sense?" is a good yardstick.

For best results with this book, I recommend that you read the chapters in the order presented, starting with the Introduction. As you read, bear in mind that no part of this book is intended as medical or dental advice, or as a substitute for that advice. Please therefore discuss your health issues, and what you learn in this book, with your attending healthcare professional(s). You'll find additional details for consumers and healthcare professionals in a special section just for book readers, which you'll find at www.HolisticMouthSolutions. com/BookBonuses.

If you're ready to turn on wellness, turn back illness, and stop one health trouble after another, *Early Sirens* will illuminate what you've been missing in order to succeed, and will show you what a painless and natural Holistic Mouth as a natural solution can do for your whole body health.

Felix Liao, DDS, MAGD, ABGD, MIABDM
Falls Church, Virginia, September, 2017

Praise for Early Sirens

"Dr. Felix Liao has now produced a wonderful expansion on his initial work, *Six-Foot Tiger, Three-Foot Cage* in his new book, *Early Sirens*. Dr. Liao is a rare heath pioneer in that he demonstrates how many dental and ultimately medical problems start with abnormalities of head and neck anatomy.

It is readily apparent from the experiences of his patients and from the scientific literature that a very large number of life-threatening diseases get their start because the oral cavity anatomy never had the proper proportions at birth. It is also apparent that pediatricians, physicians who treat adolescents, and pediatric dentists should be routinely referring children for a Holistic Mouth Checkup early-on in their lives.

Once a medical problem starts, the disease becomes the focus, and only very rarely is any thought given to helping correct the anatomic abnormalities that often feed that disease.

I offer my highest recommendation for this latest work by Dr. Liao. It should be required reading for all dentists and physicians, preferably before they graduate."

Thomas E. Levy, MD, JD,
Author of *Death by Calcium, Uninformed Consent,*
and *Hidden Epidemic: Silent Oral Infections Cause
Most Heart Attacks and Breast Cancers*

"Liao's *Early Sirens* correlates impaired mouth structures with numerous chronic symptoms and illnesses in a clear and understandable way that is appropriate for both health professionals as well as holistically-oriented individuals interested in improving their health. For millions of people, not only can insomnia and sleep apnea be successfully treated with functional oral appliances, but many other health complaints can be cured through treating the root cause—a dysfunctional airway due to crowded teeth and misaligned/ underdeveloped jaws."

Louisa L. Williams, MS. DC, ND,
Author of Radical Medicine

"Dr. Liao's *Early Sirens* brilliant connects the dots into a coherent downhill slide story from Impaired Mouth structure to airway obstruction to sleep apnea. This allows you to reverse course in time by using his most sensible Holistic Mouth Solutions."

Dr. Sherry Salartash, DDS, Alexandria, Virginia

"*Early Sirens* is not only a must read for the public, it is a must read for all health professionals."

Mark A. Breiner, DDS, Author of Whole-Body Dentistry

"There are many oral health issues that can have a significant, and negative, effect on overall health. These range from gum infection to chronic mercury poisoning from mercury released from amalgam fillings. In Dr. Felix Liao's brilliant book *Early Sirens*, he addresses a number of other important oral health issues, including root-canals, snoring, teeth grinding, and malocclusion, that can also have a severe impact on both oral and overall health. I strongly believe every patient should be evaluated for the issues he discusses in his book and once identified be treated appropriately. While written for the patient I also consider it a must read for every practicing dentist. Very well written and illustrated, it is also easy to understand, with well thought out treatment solutions. I've known Dr. Liao for many years and have a very high regard for his experience and dedication to superior whole-body health by Holistic Mouth.

I highly recommend this excellent book for anyone who sincerely wants to achieve optimal oral health and eliminate the health symptoms related to the specific oral health issues he discusses in *Early Sirens.*"

Tom McGuire, DDS,
Author of *The Poison in Your Teeth, Mercury Detoxification, and Healthy Teeth – Healthy Body.*

"Look, it's really quite simple. Any dental care professional who isn't equipped to properly diagnose Impaired Mouth Syndrome is doing a profound disservice to a significant percentage of patients. Any dental practice that isn't equipped to successfully correct the root causes of Impaired Mouth Syndrome is depriving those patients of a superior solution that can thrill and delight them like no other. If these audacious assertions don't peak your curiosity, don't read *Early Sirens*. If they do, you owe it to yourself to take this — and all of Dr. Felix Liao's books to heart... whether you're suffering from the symptoms he describes, or you're a dental professional who cares deeply about providing your patients with lasting solutions."

Dr. David Gruder, PhD,
11-Award-Winning Integrative Health Professional
& Enterprise Success Psychologist, who Radio & TV
Interview Reports Named America's Integrity Expert

"In the real world, malocclusion is wide spread. In hospitals and doctors' offices, malocclusion is under-recognized, and in the dental offices, under-treated. Jaw alignment with the Whole, and dental alignment within the jaws are just not considered, and the patient is the one who ultimately suffers. Dentistry is the only profession with the capability to help in this area and especially dentist trained in looking for the signs and symptoms that lead to disease based on compromised Airway and decreases in oxygen. Dr. Liao, has put together another great book that explains the connections and solutions for Impaired Mouth Syndrome."

Dr. Sylvester Gonzales, Round Rock, Texas

"Since learning and working with Dr. Liao, I see so many signs that I missed before and now feel I am better equipped to help my patients. Reading Early Sirens brilliantly connects the dots into a coherent downhill slide story from Impaired Mouth structure to airway obstruction to sleep apnea. This allows you to reverse course in time by using his most sensible Holistic Mouth Solutions.

Thank you for being my mentor and helping this "tooth doctor" through all of this to become a "mouth doctor". I am honored to learn from you, Dr. Liao"

Cristin MePherson-Lewis, DDS, Nashville, TN

Disclaimer

The opinions, advice and recommendations in this book are intended for a wide audience of people and are not tailored or specific to any individual needs or health conditions.

This book is not intended as a substitute for professional medical or dental advice, diagnosis, or treatment. Always seek professional medical advice from your dentist, physician or other qualified heath care provider with any questions you may have regarding a medical condition. This book is not intended to diagnose, treat or cure any disease. Significant changes in your health regime should be discussed with your health care provider.

The authors and publishers of this book make no warranty, representation, or guarantee regarding the advice given in this book, nor do they assume any liability whatsoever arising out of your use of any information or product referenced in this book.

Dedication

This book is dedicated to all patients seeking natural health and wellness who push their doctors, dentists, and all healthcare professionals to find more effective solutions at the root cause level.

Table of Contents

Introduction

The Body's Early Sirens: Critical Clues to Serious Medical-Dental Troubles Ahead

The doctor of the future will give no medicine, but will instruct his patient in the care of the human frame, in diet and in the cause and prevention of disease.

– Thomas Edison (*1903*)

If Edison's vision resonates with you as a patient, or inspires you as a healthcare professional, then this book is for you. If you have seen many doctors and tried many treatments without success, this book may also be for you.

Most Americans today have been conditioned to see doctors as fixers of failed/failing health. But a doctor's title is derived from its Latin origin - *docēre* – meaning a teacher. A doctor true to his/her title shows patients not only why health goes wrong, but also what can be done, and how to prevent it from going wrong. That's why I started my *Holistic Mouth Solutions* series — to call attention to the mouth's pivotal role in natural health and wellness.

Life at birth starts with a cry to inflate the lungs, then a feeding, followed by peaceful sleep. Repeating that pattern (minus the cry) leads to growth in childhood and health and wellness – or lack thereof – in adulthood, all the way to the final breath. It's fair to say that the mouth is a life source and a health driver, but this health driver remains largely unknown to doctors, dentists, healthcare professionals, and their patients in 2017.

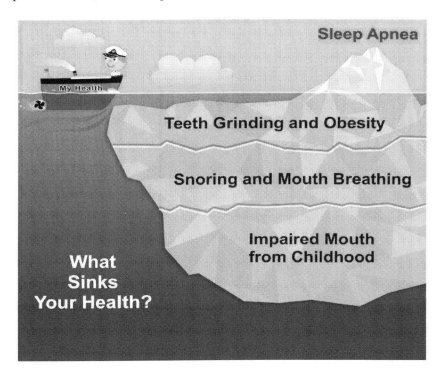

The mouth is a big part of daily life, and it does a whole lot more for us than eating, drinking, and talking. The two jaws combine with the eyes to form the face that identifies each of us, and with the cranium housing the brain to form the head as the body's command and control center. Despite its many functions, the mouth's structural form is critically missing in the care of health today.

Good health requires a well-formed mouth, and a structurally deficient mouth means health troubles. That's an organizing principle for our entire body. Many chronically ill patients live with a deformed set of jaws without their knowing, and millions more are heading toward costly health degeneration without their doctors knowing.

Most people and doctors know that poor sleep means poor health, but do you know WHY and HOW the mouth can be the anatomical source? We are talking about structure here, not diet or personal eating style. Under-developed jaws result in not only crowded teeth, but also a narrower airway that can lower life quality, raise medical and dental costs, and shorten life span, as you will see shortly.

More importantly, how can we be proactive on the nagging and catastrophic impacts on our personal health and national treasury from impaired sleep-airway-mouth?

Heart and Alzheimer's diseases, cancer, stroke, diabetes — leading killers of Americans — are adversely affected to a greater degree by sleeping with a partially-choked airway than diet, in my opinion. This deficient airway can be traced back to a structurally impaired mouth as a defective infrastructure, as we shall see ahead.

Snoring, jaw clicking, teeth grinding, chronic pain and fatigue, and the pattern of one dental problem after another are routinely ignored by the patient and overlooked by health professionals, based on my patients' experience. This book explains how and why this happens, its consequences, and – most importantly – offer real, long-term solutions to this often ignored drag on overall health and well-being.

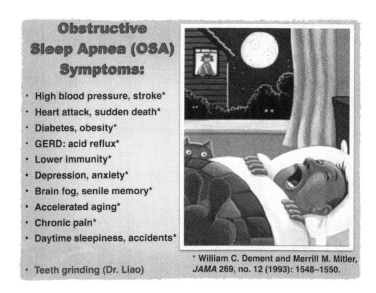

Obstructive Sleep Apnea (OSA) Symptoms:

- High blood pressure, stroke*
- Heart attack, sudden death*
- Diabetes, obesity*
- GERD: acid reflux*
- Lower immunity*
- Depression, anxiety*
- Brain fog, senile memory*
- Accelerated aging*
- Chronic pain*
- Daytime sleepiness, accidents*
- Teeth grinding (Dr. Liao)

* William C. Dement and Merrill M. Mitler, *JAMA* 269, no. 12 (1993): 1548–1550.

Holistic Mouth: Foundational to Whole Body Health

If you have already read *Six-Foot Tiger Three Foot Cage (6T3C)*, first let me thank you, and you can skip ahead to the next section, The Body's Early Sirens. This section is a summary for first-timers of the key concepts in *(6T3C)*, or if you read it and want a quick review.

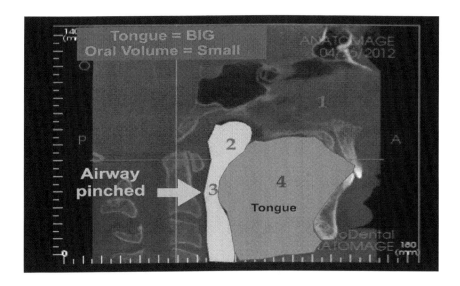

When your oral space between the two jaws is too small, the tongue is forced backward to close down airway where it becomes a life-threatening "tiger". Stating the problem this way suggests its own solution: redeveloping the undersized and misaligned jaws can provide a suitable habitat for your tongue and room for all crowded/impacted teeth, and dramatically upgrade your overall health and life quality.

Redevelopment here means changing the shape and increasing the volume of the undersized upper and lower jaws and the space between and around them, such as the nasal passage and the oral airway behind the tongue. Other new concepts and key principles that were introduced in *6T3C* include:

- A Holistic Mouth is structurally fit to support whole body health through the ABCDES: Alignment, Breathing, Circulation, Digestion, Energy, and Sleep.

- Even though an Impaired Mouth can eat, drink, and talk, its poor form disrupts the ABCDES and creates a far-ranging set of medical, dental, and mood symptoms that I named Impaired Mouth Syndrome. When an Impaired Mouth is structurally corrected, overall health improves naturally, and often dramatically.

- Holistic Mouth is a natural solution to resolve/mitigate Impaired Mouth Syndrome at the root cause level. New epigenetic oral appliances can transform an Impaired Mouth into a Holistic Mouth by activating the stem cells in the root sockets of your healthy teeth.

- WholeHealth is a holistic philosophy that integrates all the parts and systems within our mind-body-mouth into a functional Whole. In contrast, patchwork care manages symptoms at best while leaving the cause(s) untouched, and this means that new troubles can sprout up again later.

Impaired Mouth Syndrome Score

Impaired Mouth Syndrome Score©

from *Six-Foot Tiger, Three-Foot Cage*, by Dr. Felix Liao

Mouth	Score	Body	Score
Snoring, morning dry mouth	0 1	Gasping or choking in sleep	0 1
Teeth grinding, jaw clenching	0 1	Neck, shoulder, or back pain; headaches	0 1
Mouth breathing, chapped lips	0 1	Erectile dysfunction or PMS	0 1
Persistent/wandering dental sensitivity	0 1	High blood pressure, heart disease	0 1
Gum recession and/or redness	0 1	Diabetes type 2, bloating after meals	0 1
Clicking/locking jaw joints, zigzag jaw opening	0 1	Weight gain, pot belly; acid reflux	0 1
Morning headache and/or sore jaws	0 1	Daytime sleepiness, fatigue	0 1
Deep overbite or underbite (weak chin)	0 1	Senile memory, ADD/ADHD	0 1
Frequent cavities or broken/chipped teeth	0 1	Frequent colds, flu, and skin disorders	0 1
Teeth prints on the sides of the tongue	0 1	Obstructive sleep apnea from a sleep test	0 1
Bony outgrowth on palate or inside lower jaw	0 1	Stuffy/runny nose, scratchy/itchy throat	0 1
Sunken lips and reverse smile curve (sad)	0 1	Forward head: ears ahead of shoulders	0 1
History of teeth extractions for braces	0 1	Waking up to urinate more than once	0 1
Bulge under lower jaw, double chin	0 1	Large neck size (M>17, W>15)	0 1
History of lots of dental work + medical symptoms	0 1	Poor digestion and elimination	0 1
Malocclusion (crowded teeth)	0 1	Depression, anxiety, grouchiness	0 1
Total Score		Total Score	

www.HolisticMouthSolutions.com

The Body's Early Sirens

Our body works as a coordinated Whole of seamlessly integrated systems and mutually dependent parts. Our bodies pay a heavy price for Impaired Mouth Syndrome that, among other things, includes oxygen deficiency and dental angina that can kill "the nerves" inside teeth and result in much-dreaded root-canal treatments.

In my WholeHealth view, the sounds of snoring, teeth grinding, jaw clicking, and the bodily messages of chronic pain and fatigue, dental sensitivity, and the pattern of one-dental-problem-after-another, are leading indicators of bigger health troubles ahead. These symptoms are the equivalent of footprints at a crime scene that in my experience invariably leads us to the culprit of an Impaired Mouth with a clogged airway that has a wide range life-altering negative impacts that I described in *6T3C*.

My thesis of *Early Sirens* is this: teeth grinding, jaw clicking, sensitive teeth, and toothaches are early warnings from the body that it is on a downhill slide toward sleep apnea, heart disease, brain degeneration, accelerated aging, and even premature death. That makes dental visits valuable opportunities to screen for Impaired Mouth Syndrome's early clues, provided that the dentist is trained as a Holistic Mouth doctor.

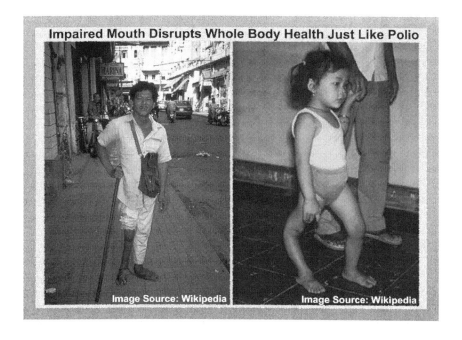

Impaired Mouth Disrupts Whole Body Health Just Like Polio

Image Source: Wikipedia

Image Source: Wikipedia

A polio-impaired leg disrupts the Whole in dramatically visible ways. An Impaired Mouth disrupts the Whole in less visible but no less dramatic ways. Our mouth ranks high in our body's organizational chart. Dysfunctions throughout our body will continue until critical wellness functions in our head and mouth are restored with better alignment and fuller development, as shown in *Six-foot Tiger, Three-foot Cage*.

The title *Early Sirens* reflects the prevention mindset built into the DNA of the dental profession. Other than sudden traumatic blows, teeth are lost only after a long progression of symptoms. Paying attention to the available clues early on allows timely interventions to stop or slow downward deterioration, dentally, orally, and systemically.

Seeing with New Eyes: Holistic Mouth Is Preventive Natural Medicine

By closely inspecting the oral-facial signs of Impaired Mouth, patients and healthcare professionals can prevent or slow the avoidable downward slide in patient health toward sleep apnea, chronic pain and fatigue, heart attack, stroke, tooth loss, memory loss, and more.

In other words, many medical, dental, and mental-mood troubles can be avoided if Impaired Mouth Syndrome can be identified early on — when teeth grinding, jaw clicking, and snoring starts, and long before the body suffers irreversible tooth loss and organ damage. All it takes is patient education and professionals training to grow some new eyes. With this in mind, let's start with a couple of questions:

- Did you wake up this morning feeling tired and wishing you could keep sleeping, or did you feel refreshed and ready to take on the new day?
- Do you rely on caffeine, sugary carbs, energy drinks, candy, or naps to cope with daytime sleepiness day after day – or wish you could?

Your answers contain messages from your body that are potential early warning signs of health troubles ahead. This Early Sirens book will decode these messages, connect the dots, and trace the trail back to the biggest overlooked cause: Impaired Mouth, featuring deficient and misaligned jaws, crowded teeth, a pinched airway, and much more. I'll provide you with evidence-based explanations and reveal painless natural solutions that have been helping many patients resolve and prevent symptoms.

Here are some additional questions for your own CSI:

- Do you snore in your sleep, or sleep with someone who does regularly?

- Do you wear a night guard to protect your teeth from grinding or a CPAP mask to cope with sleep apnea – or have been told that you should?

- Do your jaw joints click and pop when you open or close your mouth?

- Do you have chronic pain and fatigue? Depression? Anxiety?

- Do you have lingering dental sensitivities, tenderness to bite, or one dental trouble after another? Have you been told that you need dental implants or reconstruction?

- Are you living with diabetes, overweight, acid reflux, heart disease?

- Are you concerned about fuzzy memory, brain fog, or Alzheimer' disease?

Such medical, dental, and mood symptoms often stem from a structurally impaired mouth, in my experience. I'll provide you with evidence-based explanations and reveal painless natural solutions that can help many patients resolve and prevent symptoms when adopted.

Impaired Mouth Syndrome is as prevalent as it is because very few healthcare professionals are trained to look for, assess, and treat these sleep-airway-mouth connections.

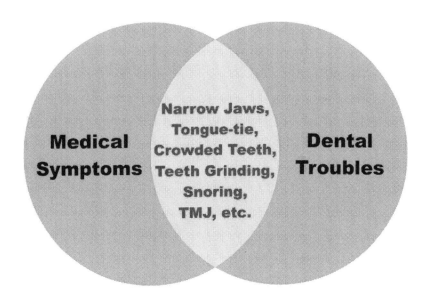

A Field Report from A Wake

Just how real is this connection? Here is an email from one of my patients:

> I had heard Dr. Liao speak on 'A Mouth Doctor's View on Natural Health and Wellness' one Saturday, and his point was about how critical an unobstructed airway is for good sleep and good health....
>
> The very next day, I attended a wake for a friend who had passed away of a heart attack. People were puzzled about his sudden death. Then they touched on how he had been struggling with sleep issues for some time and that the night he passed away, his wife awoke to the sounds of him gasping for breath.
>
> As we continued our conversation, several of my friends mentioned that they, too, had sleep and breathing issues. They started talking about their doctor recommended

CPAP machines (the device designed to force air down the constricted behind the tongue and soft palate) and how difficult it was to sleep with them in place.

I was amazed at how accurate Dr. Liao's assertions were. Our very life and breath are at risk. We need to wake up and recognize the pivotal role oral health plays in our well-being and longevity.

Don't need to wait for a wake to wake up. As one acupuncturist-homeopathic doctor told me, "I suddenly realized in the middle of your lecture that half my patients have mouth structure issues. No remedy, supplement, or magic bullet will work until sleep-airway-mouth link is restored first."

Is your mouth a health asset, or liability? Is there something you can do before you or a loved one gets to the end of that downhill slide with a serious medical condition or without your natural teeth and a huge dental bill?

My answer is YES — the earth is no longer flat in healthcare. We are in the new era of WholeHealth — you can finally re-develop the airway inside a "three-foot cage" and reopen that oxygen lifeline to reinvigorate your natural health and wellbeing instead of creating significant health problems.

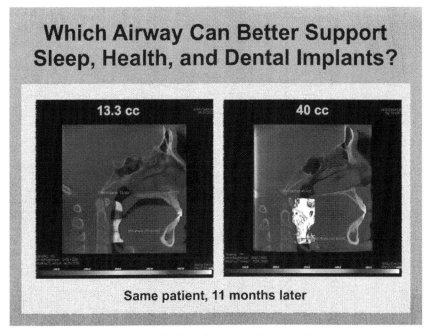

Which Airway Can Better Support Sleep, Health, and Dental Implants?

13.3 cc   40 cc

Same patient, 11 months later

*Profile view of the head's center slice, —with upper
and lower front teeth near the right edge.*

*Color Scale: white means the airway is wide open and not susceptible
to collapse during sleep; the colors toward the red zone represents
increasingly narrow airway at higher risk of collapse.*

WholeHealth vs. Fragmented Care

Good health is a narrow perch on top of a tent of;'/. inter-connected body parts and seamlessly integrated organ systems. Your mouth supports that perch – a state known medically as homeostasis.

Good health starts to slide downhill when the mouth is structurally impaired and the airway pinched. An Impaired Mouth triggers the first domino's fall toward inevitable health decline through the gradual development of sleep apnea.

Conventional healthcare uses "band-aids" attempts to manage the diverse symptoms of Impaired Mouth Syndrome. Examples of this include antibiotics overuse, opioid dependency without considering structural realignment of head-jaws-spine, and treating neck pain without considering how a bad bite might be creating that pain — see chapters 8-12.

Instead, WholeHealth investigates the root causes of said symptoms to naturally restore the Whole back to homeostasis as much as possible — see chapter 9 for a more detailed discussion.

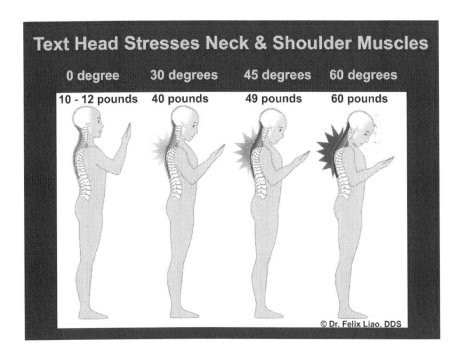

WholeHealth sees all parts of your body are connected without department lines. Trigger points refer pain from the source to a distant site. Trigger points in the neck and shoulder muscles can be controlled to mitigate the need for root-canal treatment — see chapter 8.

WholeHealth reflects the holographic truth throughout the body. The oxygen deficiency from pinched airway inside Impaired Mouth is bad for both the heart AND the teeth. Erectile dysfunction is a red flag for circulatory health decline. So is the pattern of one root-canal treatment after another — it may just be the dental version of heart angina.

WholeHealth's recognition of Dental Angina has led to new ways of avoiding root-canal treatment by reversing certain toothaches and dental sensitivities without the usual drills and pills — see chapter 11.

WholeHealth is also a platform on which doctors and therapists of all types can collaborate to help patients restore and maintain whole body health — see Tandem Treatment in chapter 13 and Cranio-sacral Therapy in Chapter 18.

In a nutshell, good health requires restorative sleep, which in turn requires a Holistic Mouth. It's time for WholeHealth teamwork.

From Illness to Wellness

What's the difference between illness and wellness? Energy in the body's "gas tank" would be my one-phrase answer.

How do you fill that energy tank? Eat right, exercise, balance work with relaxation, and get a good night's sleep. It is not that complicated to understand, but it's not delivered in America's healthcare in 2017. Why? Going to sleep with the tongue blocking your airway is a much-overlooked health blocker and bank breaker.

In contrast, WholeHealth wellness starts with ensuring quality sleep by making sure your sleep-airway-mouth link works properly. A wide-open airway is the pipeline to strong heart, high-octane brain, aging well, and thus a top prize in healthcare.

Your body knows how to run and how to fix itself far better than all your doctors added together. I believe the full healing power of God/ Nature is downloaded into the body during deep sleep.

As far as your heart, brain, and teeth are concerned, deep sleep is the only meaningful health insurance.

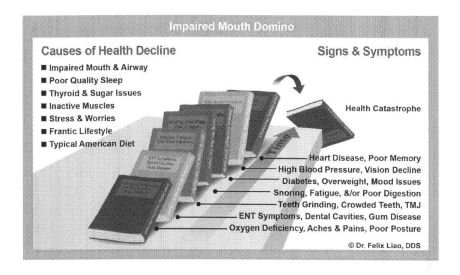

Holistic Mouth: Simple Concept and Powerful Solution

"I wish I had known about your Holistic Mouth earlier!" New patients often say to me. "How come my doctors and dentists never told me about this?"

Impaired Mouth Syndromes and Holistic Mouth Solutions are brand new concepts and practices. Few health professionals are aware that a structurally underdeveloped mouth (featuring deep overbite, weak chin, sunken mid-face, narrow jaws, crowded teeth, double chin, and so on) can be the source of many medical, dental, mood, and life quality problems.

Even fewer know how to solve them at the source. It's not their fault. Odds are that the mouth was not part of their training and thus remains missing in their thinking.

Nonetheless, science is evolving, the "old box" is expanding, and better outcome are coming from WholeHealth thinking. WholeHealth is a unifying platform for clinical collaboration among all health professionals, employers, and insurers to help patients stay healthy and productive.

It is time to start identifying and correcting the source of disease instead of managing its downstream symptoms. It is time to listen to your body's "early sirens." Paying attention to these indicators can potentially save you from health and financial catastrophes later, as the cases ahead will show.

Holistic Mouth is a simple concept and a powerful solution. The best natural medicine is refreshing sleep, and the best health insurance is a wide-open airway. This is the foundational principle of Holistic Mouth Solutions™.

Let's see what Holistic Mouth as a natural solution has done for my patients, and can do for you.

Chapter 1

Snoring — Health Risks Iceberg Ahead and What Lurks Between and Below

Even snoring, a phenomenon often thought of by those affected as benign, is associated with poor prognosis in individuals who are at risk for cardiovascular disease and also can increase risk of stroke.

– William C. Dement, MD, PhD, and Merrill M. Mitler, PhD [1]

"Either go to sleep on the couch or to see Dr. Felix — that's what my wife said." T.P. answered after I asked this new patient how I could help him.

Three months later, his wife and mother of their four young children emailed me:

I am glad to not be waking up in the night in a panic because my husband sounds like he's choking to death. I am thankful for your appliance for my husband. It is healing *my* adrenal fatigue. After he had it for one week, I was feeling like a new person!

Suffice it to say, it helped T.P., too.

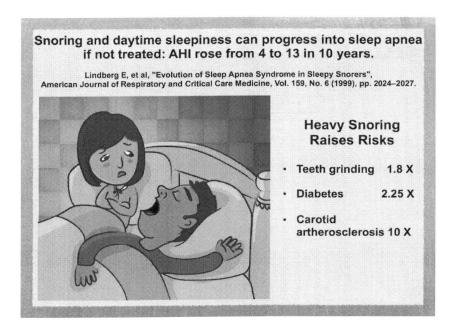

Snoring and daytime sleepiness can progress into sleep apnea if not treated: AHI rose from 4 to 13 in 10 years.

Lindberg E, et al, "Evolution of Sleep Apnea Syndrome in Sleepy Snorers", American Journal of Respiratory and Critical Care Medicine, Vol. 159, No. 6 (1999), pp. 2024–2027.

Heavy Snoring Raises Risks

- Teeth grinding   1.8 X
- Diabetes   2.25 X
- Carotid artherosclerosis 10 X

Snoring: More Than an Annoyance

Snoring is more than an annoyance to the sleep partner. The noise is from the vibration of air rushing over the soft palate, tonsils, and throat tissues. Sometimes snoring can be just pure and simple noise from mouth breathing during sleep. Other times, it can be a symptom of sleep apnea and an early siren of health troubles ahead. This is especially the case if:

- Snoring is a nightly occurrence for years
- The snorer is overweight

- Teeth grinding, jaw clenching is present — no noise is needed
- Snoring is accompanied by witnessed evens of stopped breathing, choking, gasping, or waking up in a panic
- Morning grogginess and daytime sleepiness, which can be suggestive of sleep apnea.

What is the best way to tell the difference between benign and dangerous snoring? A thorough health history, a doctor consultation, and possibly a sleep test. Even without those, there are four common oral-facial features that suggest airway obstruction as a potential problem, and T.P. exhibited all of them.

- Backward head tilt and Forward neck extension so the ear opening is well ahead of the shoulder point. T.P.'s head posture suggested airway struggle, and a CT scan confirmed that his airway was less than half of low normal in volume, and 20% in width.

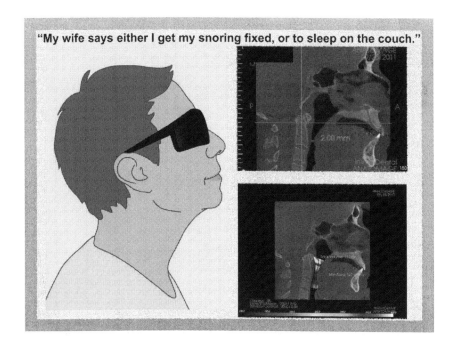

"My wife says either I get my snoring fixed, or to sleep on the couch."

- Liao's Sign: upper lip is flat or curled in profile view. A positive Liao's sign implicates a less than optimal airway until proven otherwise. Yet the absence of Liao's sign does not mean all is well.

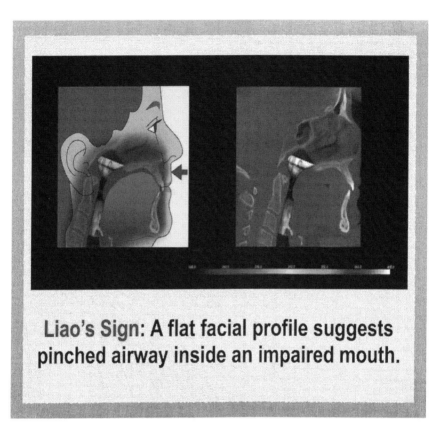

Liao's Sign: A flat facial profile suggests pinched airway inside an impaired mouth.

- Uvula not visible with the mouth open and the tongue inside the lower dental arch (Friedman Tongue Position Test). The less you can see the uvula (the tissue that hangs at the back of your mouth, above your throat), tonsils, and soft palate – because they appear blocked by the tongue – the higher the sleep apnea risk.

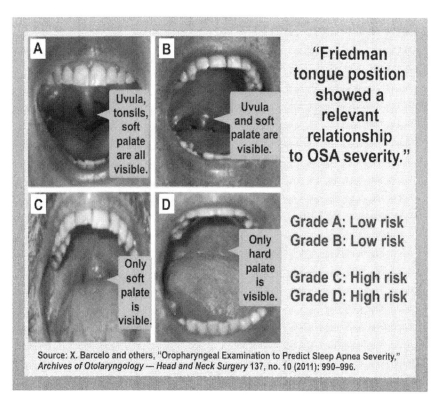

A. Uvula, tonsils, soft palate are all visible.

B. Uvula and soft palate are visible.

C. Only soft palate is visible.

D. Only hard palate is visible.

"Friedman tongue position showed a relevant relationship to OSA severity."

Grade A: Low risk
Grade B: Low risk

Grade C: High risk
Grade D: High risk

Source: X. Barcelo and others, "Oropharyngeal Examination to Predict Sleep Apnea Severity," *Archives of Otolaryngology — Head and Neck Surgery* 137, no. 10 (2011): 990–996.

- Crowded lower front teeth; this is a reflection of deficient maxilla (upper jaw) that is the cardinal feature of an Impaired Mouth, as mentioned in Chapter 12 of *Six-foot Tiger Three-foot Cage*. Crowded teeth mean smaller jaws which in turn drives the tongue into the throat.

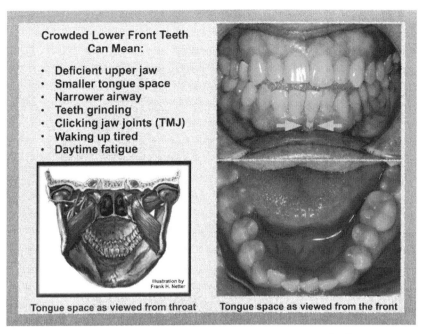

Top left: arrows point to gum recession as a result of push-pull action between tongue and lips.

Snoring can be the result of partial airway obstruction, which, over time, can run up a serious oxygen debt that can be hard on your heart, brain, and yes, teeth. A firm stand by their sleep partner can potentially save a snorer's vital organs and even their life

More Energy: Evidence of Airway and Sleep Improvement

I told T.P. of his options: (A) sleep with his lower jaw held forward with a mandibular advancement appliance that does not change his existing bad bite, or (B) wear a set of upper and lower expanders for adults mRNA Appliance™ — a set of upper and lower expanders for adults that works while holding the lower jaw in a forward position during sleep – to reopen and redevelop his deficient upper and lower jaws during sleep. [2]

T.P. opted for the latter and just a few weeks later reported, "Since I started using the appliance, I've had more energy, and my wife really appreciates that I'm sleeping through the night without snoring, and she's getting better rest, too."

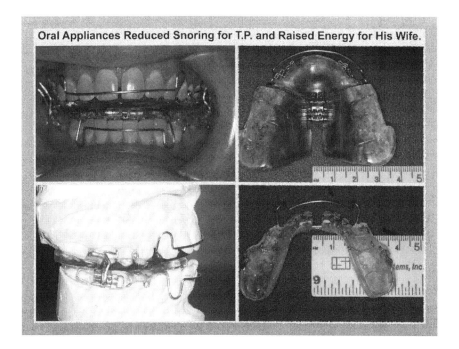

Oral Appliances Reduced Snoring for T.P. and Raised Energy for His Wife.

Snoring Harms Two

Snoring harms the health of both the snorer and the sleep partner. It is one big reason why 23% of couples sleep apart and new homes are trending toward two master bedrooms.

Conversely, treating the snorer helps the sleep partner, reports a Mayo Clinic study: "Elimination of snoring and OSA improved the quality of the bed partner's sleep and symptoms more than the snorer, including tiredness, headaches, and poor sleep." [3] The same study found that, over eight hours, sleep partners gained an extra 62 minutes of sleep with a 13% gain in sleep efficiency (percent of time the brain is actually asleep versus total time in bed). That's why Mrs. T.P. felt so much better.

I enjoy treating snoring because one set of oral appliances can help two people, and the whole family. If you are prevention-oriented, then it is prudent to consider snoring as a leading indicator of possible medical, dental, and brain troubles ahead.

Habitual Snoring: A Loud Warning of Health Troubles Ahead

Snoring is mouth breathing, which comes with many health and social hazards. "Dragon breath" and "cotton mouth" in the morning means the gums and teeth are deprived of saliva's immune protection.

More importantly, snoring reflects airway obstruction and therefore health troubles ahead. "Snoring seems to be a potential determinant of risk of ischaemic heart disease [blocked coronary artery] and stroke", concludes a 1987 study published in the British Medical Journal. [4] In that study "there were no cases of stroke among the non-snorers", whereas the risk for frequent habitual snorers is 2.38 times."

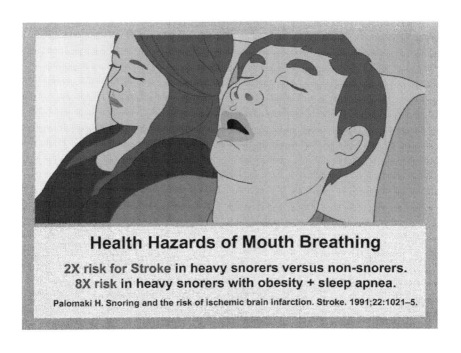

Health Hazards of Mouth Breathing

2X risk for Stroke in heavy snorers versus non-snorers.
8X risk in heavy snorers with obesity + sleep apnea.

Palomaki H. Snoring and the risk of ischemic brain infarction. Stroke. 1991;22:1021–5.

Habitual snoring (more than half the time) is a loud message from the body to investigate a clogged airway inside an impaired mouth. That's because snoring can be important in stroke and Alzheimer's prevention — two of the most expensive diseases. The two carotid arteries, one on each side of the neck, supply blood to the face, mouth, eyes, and front half of the brain. They can also bring blood clots to cause stroke and serious vision complications.

Left unrecognized and untreated, snoring can progress into sleep apnea. [5] This where a dentist trained as a doctor of Holistic Mouth can be of great service in early detection and intervention at 6-month checkup time. The evidence in the next section points to the wisdom of identifying deficient airway and an Impaired Mouth early.

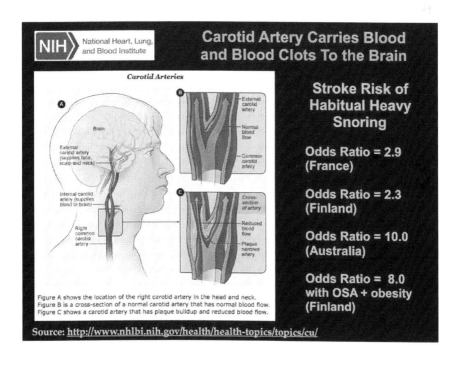

Carotid Artery Carries Blood and Blood Clots To the Brain

NIH — National Heart, Lung, and Blood Institute

Carotid Arteries

Stroke Risk of Habitual Heavy Snoring

Odds Ratio = 2.9 (France)

Odds Ratio = 2.3 (Finland)

Odds Ratio = 10.0 (Australia)

Odds Ratio = 8.0 with OSA + obesity (Finland)

Figure A shows the location of the right carotid artery in the head and neck. Figure B is a cross-section of a normal carotid artery that has normal blood flow. Figure C shows a carotid artery that has plaque buildup and reduced blood flow.

Source: http://www.nhlbi.nih.gov/health/health-topics/topics/cu/

More Evidence of Harm from Habitual Snoring

How does habitual snoring harm your health? Here are just a few answers from science:

- Snoring is associated with an 8 times greater risk of stroke in the presence of obesity, excessive daytime sleepiness, and sleep apnea [6].

- "Habitual snoring carries a significant risk factor for stroke," reports a 2009 study from France. The authors suggest "inquiring about habitual snoring should become a routine practice, especially among older male patients with arterial hypertension, and specific preventive measures should be instituted at an earlier stage." [7]

- A habitual snorer has more than twice the chance of having a stroke than a non-snorer. A study from Finland found that "the odds ratio of snoring for brain infarction [stroke] was 2.13." [8]

- "Heavy snoring significantly increases the risk of carotid [artery] atherosclerosis, with an odds ratio of 10.5, independent of OSA severity," according to a 2008 Australian study. [9]

- Regular snorers have 2.25 times the risk for type 2 diabetes, while part-time snorers have 1.48 times the risk, according to a study from the Harvard School of Public Health. [10]

- "Most often, palatal surgery alters sound characteristics of snoring, but is no cure for this disorder," according to a 2010 report from Belgium's Ghent University. [11]

- "… heavy and habitual snoring represents a risk factor for the cardiovascular system." A 1980 Italian study found 24 percent of males and nearly 14 percent of females were habitual snorers. Rates skyrocketed to more than 60 percent of men and 40 percent of women in their early 60s. Habitual snorers were more likely to be overweight: 54 percent vs. 34 percent. [12]

- Snoring amounts to mouth breathing, which aggravates oxygen deficiency by making it more tightly bound to the red blood cells through the Bohr effect. [13]

Snoring Treatment with Oral Appliances

Dentistry is evolving from drill-and-fill to health and well-being starting with the mouth and airway. Dentists trained as doctors of Holistic Mouth are in a strategic position to make a powerful difference in their patients' whole body health.

Oral appliance therapy is recommended for snoring, says the American Academy of Sleep Medicine in its 2015 update:

1. We recommend that sleep physicians prescribe oral appliances, rather than no therapy, for adult patients who request treatment of primary snoring (without obstructive sleep apnea). (STANDARD)
2. When oral appliance therapy is prescribed by a sleep physician for an adult patient with obstructive sleep apnea, we suggest that a qualified dentist use a custom, titratable [adjustable] appliance over non-custom oral devices. [14]

Age Is Not a Factor: The Case of D.W.

About six months after Mrs. D.W.'s husband started oral appliance therapy, she said, "My 67-year-old husband used to snore every night and keep me awake — it was very loud and annoying. He stopped snoring after oral appliance therapy, and I am very grateful."

For his part, Mr. D.W. said, "Wearing the appliance is no trouble at all, and it's helped cut down my snoring to almost nothing. It stays in all night, and it feels natural to have it in. I've gotten more energy and can do a lot during the day, and I feel really good."

Snoring should be treated seriously because it often represents partial airway obstruction resulting in part from having the tongue as a "six-foot tiger" inside a mouth that offers only a "three-foot cage".

Epigenetic orthopedic appliances give us a way to redevelop a deficient maxilla (upper jaw) and widen the airway, even in adults. They work by stimulating stem cells inside the tooth sockets so the airway can be reshaped. Those stem cells respond predictably.

Age is not a factor as long as sound teeth are present in all four quadrants of both dental arches.

Holistic Mouth Nuggets

- The trio of teeth grinding, waking up tired, and habitual snoring can represent the start of health's downhill slide in adults.

- Snoring is readily treated with a new breed of epigenetic orthopedic oral appliances that can open up the oral airway behind the tongue and the soft palate. And treatment improves the health not just of the snorer but their sleep partner, as well.

- Assessing the cause of snoring is an opportunity to screen for Impaired Mouth Syndrome and the oral-systemic effects of blocked airway.

Chapter 2

The Most Overlooked Key to Health and Performance: Sleep-Airway-Mouth Synergy

Sleep allows your body to repair and rebuild. Deep sleep is a great way to neutralize stress hormones. Stress increases fluid retention — you can gain two pounds in body fluids just from one night of poor sleep due to stress.

– Dr. Joseph Mercola [1]

How many days a week do you wake up feeling refreshed and ready to go? Among my patients, the answer ranges from "once or twice a week" to "once a month" to "never."

Last night's sleep sets this morning's mood and drives today's productivity. We humans are endowed with a natural ability to tell who has not had a good night's sleep with one look. Poor quality sleep undermines overall health through the next decade and beyond, especially in teeth grinders and snorers.

Your body's downhill slide comes with many warnings of bigger health troubles ahead — if you and your healthcare professionals know how to read and listen to them. Blood pressure and overweight are common examples. You can ignore the early warnings until disaster strikes, or you can pay attention to the unsettling sounds of snoring, sleep apnea, jaw clicking, chronic pains and fatigue by asking "Why?", and then asking your body, "What are you trying to say to me?"

Effective corrective or preventive action requires an understanding of the why behind the bodily response. Before we go there, it is helpful to have a sleep overview to educate you in how to give sleep its rightful place in your daily life.

In Your Control: Four Lifestyle Factors + Sleep

Cardiovascular disease (CVD) is America's leading cause of death. Reducing its risk is not rocket science. "Sufficient sleep and adherence to all four traditional healthy lifestyle factors was associated with lower CVD risk. When sufficient sleep duration was added to the traditional lifestyle factors, the risk of CVD was further reduced," reports a 2014 Dutch study in the *European Journal of Preventive Cardiology.* [2]

Those four traditional healthy lifestyle factors are: 1) no smoking, 2) moderate alcohol consumption, 3) exercise three and a half hours or more each week, and 4) eating a Mediterranean diet.

The finding: habitually following those four habits reduced fatal cardiovascular disease by 67%. That reduction jumped to an 83% if you add sufficient sleep (seven hours or more each day) to the mix.

It's particularly telling that all four traditional lifestyle factors AND sleep all have to do with your mouth!

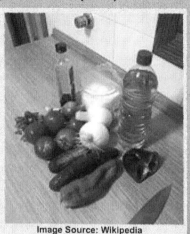

**Mediterranean Diet (MeDi)
Lowers Risks of Developing
Mild Cognitive Impairement (MCI)**

- More MeDi => lower MCI risks

- 17% lower risk for MCI in middle 1/3 vs. lowest third of MeDi adherence

- 28% lower risk for MCI in highest-1/3

- More MeDi => lower risk of MCI conversion to Alzheimer's disease

- 45% and 48% lower risk for MCI => Alzheimer's in mid-1/3 and highest 1/3, respectively, vs. lowest 1/3.

- Scarmeas N, et al, Arch Neurol. 2009 Feb; 66(2): 216–225.

Image Source: Wikipedia

The Mediterranean Lifestyle

Would the same Mediterranean diet eaten American style, i.e. picked up from a drive-through and eaten on the fly, yield the same health benefits? It's not likely, because eating, digesting, and absorbing does not mix well with stress and rush.

Slow pace, long stretch, and amiable socializing are integral parts of the Mediterranean diet. Here's what my patient Maria from Spain's Catalan region says,

"Our diet is rich in fresh fruits and vegetables, eaten in-season only. We ate lots of fish and lambs that has never had injections. Our way of life is a light breakfast between 7-9 am, a full lunch between 1-3 pm with a 20-minute siesta, a light dinner between 7-9 pm, and in bed by midnight. The average lifespan is about 95-100."

A slower mouth style is part of the Mediterranean lifestyle. And just like your diet, the health driver called sleep is in your control.

What time do you usually go to bed? How many times do you wake up overnight and when? Violation of our body's circadian rhythm (day-night cycle) has definite consequences on total health. Unfortunately, sleep has taken a backseat because the internet never sleeps.

Going to sleep and waking up consistently around a certain time is good for your health, as viewed through the lens of both modern science and Traditional Chinese Medicine.

Ying/Night Time is Restorative Time

Ying-Yang balance and cycling (from day to night and then night to day) are the foundation of Traditional Chinese Medicine (TCM). Health in the TCM view is a state of dynamic balance that is subject to external elements (weather, seasons, social atmosphere, work and home environments), as well as emotions, organs, and your internal circadian rhythm. In other words, you are different every day and every season and from hour to hour based on these factors.

Briefly, *Yang* means "sun", daytime, and energy expenditure. It also corresponds to Western medicine's sympathetic nervous system, including the fight-or-flight stress response.

Ying, on the other hand, means "shade", night, or sunset to sunrise time, and energy regeneration. It corresponds to Western medicine's parasympathetic nervous system, which deals with rest, relaxation, and energy recharge for bodily repair.

The Ying-Yang symbol thus embodies the *circadian rhythm* to which the human brain is hardwired. The sun peaks at midday, when there is minimal shadow, which then gradually lengthens while the sun fades until the dark shade peaks at night. The Yang light thus fades into Ying, which then fades into Yang at sunrise. Sleep recharges the body's "batteries", and that energy is spent the next day.

For most of my patients, the problem is too much Yang and too little Ying. This robs them of precious time to recover and regenerate from daily wear and tear.

The Body Clock in TCM

Traditional Chinese Medicine considers the internal organs and systems in terms of twelve main meridians, each of which peaks in its energy during a two-hour span each day. So, our internal body follows a clock based on the day-night cycle, the circadian rhythm. The organ-meridians connection that govern energy regeneration and bodily relaxation is listed from 7 pm to 7 am on the TCM body clock. A concise summary is available online from Naturopathic by Nature. [3]

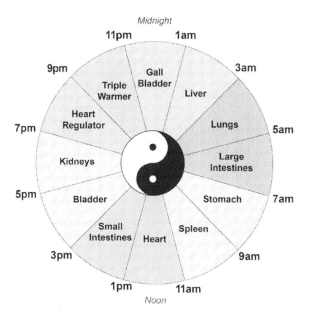

Chinese Medicine Body Clock

Note that the hours of sleep from 11 pm to 7 am involve the organs devoted to internal "house-cleaning," to detoxification and emotional release: gallbladder (toxins and grief), liver (pollutants, medications, anger), lung (breathing, sadness), colon (excretion, an overly critical/judgmental attitude).

Sustainable Health Through Nightly Renewal

While aging is inevitable, the best aging-well strategy is to maintain health in a Ying-Yang balance of energy expenditure and regeneration. In that light, let's check your daily life:

- What percentage of each 24-hour day are you in Yang, or stress mode?
- What time do you go to bed?
- What is the quality and quantity of your sleep?
- Is your body's Ying-Yang energy in balance? Where is it deficient?

The time to pay attention is not when you collapse from exhaustion, but throughout the day, and particularly after work. Sit down, relax, ease into the Ying half of the day. Make a conscious effort to designate the hours from sunset to sunrise to regenerate energy. Set an alarm to turn away from the internet and TV.

Your body is programmed to make it day after day and year after year, but only if the daily wear and tear is renewed from nightly repair and regeneration.

Sleep: Downtime or Active Time?

While your outer body may be resting during sleep, your interior body is actually quite busy. Sleep is an active time for the internal health maintenance crew — psycho-neuro-hormone-immune-detox systems — to repair and renew the body for the next day. You may wake up feeling refreshed and ready to go, or you may wake up tired and not wanting to get out of bed. The differences depend in part on

- Your overall health – where you are in health's downhill slide.

- Your recent mental-emotional state and your stress management style. Some people has a worrying or racing mind that distresses their nervous system.

- Your sleep hygiene – when you eat dinner (and how much); when you retire; total darkness; a comfortable environment; a quiet sleep partner; and so on.

- Your sleep efficiency (time asleep divided by time in bed), sleep duration, and amount of deep sleep.

- An uninterrupted supply of oxygen through an unobstructed airway.

Conversely, fighting airway obstruction to stay alive night after night for years means chronic stress to the body and excessive exposure to cortisol. Cortisol is a stress hormone that can, when over-activated, raise the risk of "anxiety, depression, digestive problems, heart disease, weight gain, insulin resistance, and memory and concentration impairment", according to Mayo Clinic. [4]

Let's take a look at some important ways in which sleep impacts your health and well-being – and what you can do to get a better night's sleep.

Sleep Strengthens Your Immune System

"Go to sleep" is the standard advice whenever you get sick. The body knows how to recover after sleep without an instructional manual — provided the airway is not obstructed.

A 2010 study from Germany concluded that growth hormones and prolactin (another tissue-building hormone) peak during night and are enhanced by sleep. At the same time, sympathetic tone (stress response) and cortisol (a stress hormone) are down during sleep. More, circulating naive T cells (fresh immune cells for detecting "bad guys" new to the immune data bank) and "killer" white blood cells and IL-10 (an anti-inflammatory marker) peak during the day. [5]

Infections and cancer win when oxygen levels and immune functions are down, and sleep plays a key role. A Wisconsin study shows cancer mortality is actually higher in direct proportion sleep apnea severity by 2-5 times. [6]

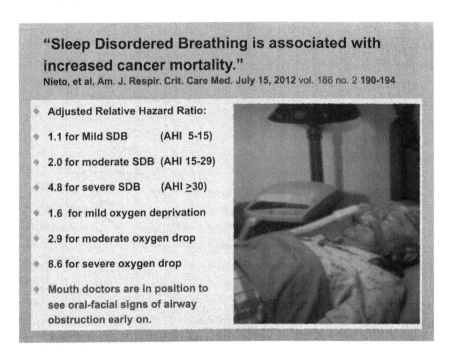

"Sleep Disordered Breathing is associated with increased cancer mortality."
Nieto, et al, Am. J. Respir. Crit. Care Med. July 15, 2012 vol. 186 no. 2 190-194

♦ Adjusted Relative Hazard Ratio:
♦ 1.1 for Mild SDB   (AHI 5-15)
♦ 2.0 for moderate SDB (AHI 15-29)
♦ 4.8 for severe SDB   (AHI ≥30)
♦ 1.6 for mild oxygen deprivation
♦ 2.9 for moderate oxygen drop
♦ 8.6 for severe oxygen drop
♦ Mouth doctors are in position to see oral-facial signs of airway obstruction early on.

Sleep is divided into two distinct states: REM (rapid eye movement) and NREM (non-REM). After an acute infection, there is more time spent in slow-wave (NREM) sleep and often a reduction of time spent in REM sleep. [7] That's why you don't feel great despite more sleep while fighting a cold.

It is now recognized that both infection-associated sleep and spontaneous sleep are regulated, in part, by immune mediators called *cytokines*. [8] Sleep deprivation reduces immunity and resistance to infection. [9]

Total sleep deprivation and chronic deep sleep (NREM) deprivation or interruption in rats produces a "reliable syndrome" that includes lethal infection, debilitated appearance and skin lesions, increased food intake, weight loss, increased energy expenditure, higher blood norepinephrine (stress hormone), decreased body temperature during the late stages of deprivation and decreased blood thyroxine (thyroid hormone), reported a study from the University of Chicago. [10]

In short, your immune system does a lot of maintenance work while you sleep. Sleep strengthens the immune system, which makes it a problem that the average sleep time of Americans is shorter than it used to be. Working or staying up too late watching TV or surfing online undermines your immune system.

Go to bed by 11pm with no electronic devices nearby and let your immune system do its thing. If you don't wake up feeling refreshed more than five or six days a week, seek help. Poor quality sleep can mean serious health troubles ahead.

The Sleep-Mood Connections

The brain runs on oxygen, and its demand for oxygen does not go down while you sleep. Mood disorders and poor memory can result from oxygen deprivation to the brain, among other factors such as the typical American diet [11] and chronic stress with cortisol as a marker [12].

"Frequent snorting/stopping breathing was associated with probable major depression," reports a 2012 study. [13]

Sleep and Mood Disorders

Source: HealthySleep.Med.Harvard.edu

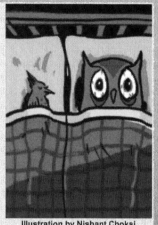

- 1/3 - 1/2 of pts with chronic sleep problems have mood disorders

- Insomnia = 20X risk for anxiety

- Insomnia = 10X risk for depression

- Difficulty sleeping is sometimes the first symptom of depression

- "People who have problems with sleep are at increased risk for developing emotional disorders, depression, and anxiety." Dr. Lawrence Epstein, Medical Director of Harvard Sleep Health Centers

Illustration by Nishant Choksi

The brain is critically dependent on oxygen. It makes sense to check for sleep apnea and airway obstruction in cases of depression. Yet in today's health care system, little attention is given to oxygen's role in mental health. Instead, antidepressants rank among the top three most prescribed therapeutic classes in doctor office visits, along with pain killers and cholesterol lowering drugs, according to CDC [14].

There are a number of hormones and neurotransmitters that are also affected by sleep. For instance, *melatonin* is made from tyrosine when the body is in the relaxed, parasympathetic mode. Its name comes from the Greek word for the color black, suggesting that it has to do with the night part of the circadian rhythm to which the human brain is wired. Being relaxed is the key for melatonin release and sleep induction.

Melatonin is a sleep hormone with powerful anti-inflammatory and free-radical scavenger functions in the brain. [15] It is made from serotonin, the feel-good neurotransmitter and helps keep the brain clean. It is secreted by the pineal gland deep in the brain following day-night cycles – another reason to respect the body's need for darkness, and go to sleep no later than 11pm.

Serotonin is negatively affected by sleep deprivation. A 2010 study from the Netherlands found that depression from insufficient sleep results from desensitization of serotonin receptors in the brain. When rats were restricted to four hours of sleep, it led to serotonin receptor desensitization in eight days. Even with unrestricted sleep afterward, the receptor took seven days to normalize. [16]

Histamine is responsible for wakefulness. (That's why drowsiness is a side effect of antihistamines.) Histamine regulates the sleep-wake cycle through light entering the eyes. There is a high release of histamine during waking hours, and it stops during rapid-eye-movement (REM) and non-rapid-eye-movement (NREM) sleep.[17] So, keep your bedroom as dark as possible. Consider installing blackout blinds whenever possible.

Dopamine also plays a role in the sleep-wake cycle. Interestingly, this neurotransmitter is out of balance in individuals with Parkinson's disease and schizophrenia – deficient in the former, excessive in the latter. A 2006 study from Duke reported that both conditions involve sleep disturbances. [18]

Bottom line: regular and healthy sleep routine can head off depression and may prevent neurological conditions.

Changing Your Sleep for the Better

Getting to bed early and getting enough deep sleep, along with eating right for your health, are crucial parts of lifestyle modification. A 2013 study reviewed 23 trials and 11,085 randomized patients: "The evidence confirms the benefits of lifestyle modification programs – over and above benefits achieved by routine clinical care alone." [19]

In other words, YOU adopting a healthy lifestyle, including sufficient quality and hours of sleep, trumps what your doctor can do for you.

Many patients wearing oral sleep appliances fail to change these parts of their life and then come in wondering why they don't feel better. I recommend that you review the tips discussed above and make a list to discuss with your doctors. What you do for your own health every day and every night can be powerful and effective natural medicine.

Just as daily brushing and flossing is essential for dental health, so nightly sleep is pivotal for total health. Both are your responsibility as the owner-operator of your body.

Signs of Quality Sleep Working: This Author's Experience

Waking up feeling refreshed and relaxed, I'd give myself a few minutes to luxuriate under the cover and wait for my mind "show up". Here's what often happens:

- A new and smarter solution to a knotty problem from yesterday would present itself, and I'd smile.

- A mental tickler would appear and say, "remember you said last night that wanted this done today?" I'd nod in appreciation.

- A more concise summary or accurate subtitle would suggest itself for this book, and I'd get out of bed happily.

Holistic Mouth Nuggets:

- Your best tomorrow comes from a great sleep tonight. Students and working adults alike need sufficient deep sleep to learn, retain, and perform. Poor quality sleep can mean serious health troubles ahead.

- A regular and healthy sleep routine can head off depression. Chronic shortage of deep sleep can reduce memory and immunity, and possibly reduce thyroid function.

- What you do for your own health every day and every night can be powerful natural medicine. If you don't wake up feeling refreshed more than five or six days a week, seek help.

Chapter 3

Teeth Grinding — The Inside Story of Sleep Bruxing Airway Disorder

Sleep bruxism is common in the general population. It has numerous consequences, which are not limited to dental or muscular problems.

– Maurice M. Ohayon, MD [1]

Teeth grinding never made sense to me. Why would the body choose to mutilate its hardest asset? The short answer: there is no choice when the airway is in need or resuscitation during sleep. Like a canary in the coal mine with impending trouble, teeth grinding should be taken seriously as a leading indicator of potential medical, dental, and brain troubles ahead.

"My eleven-year old son has been grinding his teeth ever since he had teeth," a new patient named Gerri said. I can identify with her as a parent, because I still remember that that wall-rattling sound from my son's bed room in the other corner of my house 30 years ago. I felt powerless as a dad and his dentist.

You're about to learn what took me a career to discover: Teeth grinding cannot be solved from within the silo of "teeth and teeth-only". Still, I wish I could have helped my son's teeth grinding.

"What can be done?" Gerri asked, her face full of loving concern. But before we get to treatment in the next chapter, let's understand the *WHY* behind this phenomenon.

Teeth Grinding Is Now Sleep Bruxing

Teeth grinding is not just a dental problem. In the WholeHealth view, teeth grinding reflects a health-harming process and even life-threatening struggle inside the body.

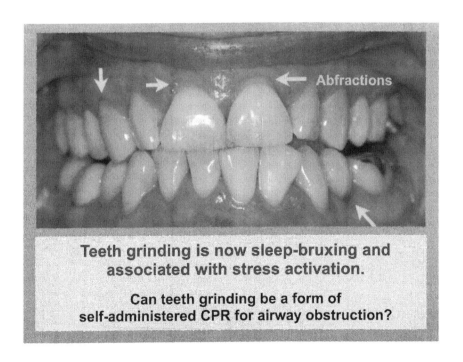

Teeth grinding is now sleep-bruxing and associated with stress activation.

Can teeth grinding be a form of self-administered CPR for airway obstruction?

The medical term for teeth grinding is now *sleep bruxing*. "Bruxing" comes from a Greek word meaning "to gnash" – and it comes with many consequences, as the opening quote points out.

A comprehensive guide on dental sleep medicine states, "Patients with sleep bruxing need to be screened for other co-morbid medical conditions (e.g., SDB [sleep-disordered breathing], insomnia, ADHD [attention deficit hyperactivity disorder], depression, mood disorders, and GERD [gastro-esophageal reflux disease] before undertaking any treatment approach, especially pharmacotherapy [medications]." [2]

Sleep bruxing/teeth grinding is the greatest source of tooth structure loss among my new patients, nearly all of whom have no cavities or gum disease. They eat organic, exercise, take supplements, and yet they often wake up tired, feel sleepy during the day, depressed, or anxious. More than 90% of the time, their teeth show matching wear facets – a telltale sign of bruxing.

Why? Because the evolved view sees bruxing as a reaction to airway obstruction during sleep and a form of CPR to alleviate oxygen crisis without giving up sleep. Teeth grinding is a higher "DEFCON" warning than snoring, in my opinion.

Code Blue!! — The Inside Story of Sleep Bruxing

Bruxing may be a survival tactic in reaction to a life-or-death crisis from airway obstruction during sleep. Obstructive sleep apnea (OSA) is a condition in which breathing stops due to the collapse of the airway between the back of the soft palate (Zone2 in the diagram below) and the back of the tongue (Zone 3), and the severity is measured in terms of the number of apnea, or absence of breathing.

Upper Airway Spaces

- **Zone 1: Nasal cavity**

- **Zone 2: Nasal pharynx**

- **Zone 3: Oral pharynx**

- **Zone 4: Oral cavity**

Good airway needs good form: ALL four zones wide and open.

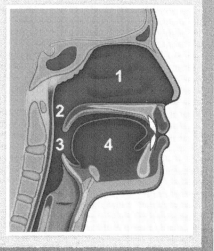

If you don't have dizziness when you stand up from lying down, you can try this little test: Open the timer app in your smartphone. Breathe normally, then after inhaling, zip your lips and pinch your nose shut so no air goes in or out, and start the timer. After 10 seconds, lift your hand off and breathe through your nose.

Are you glad you can take that next breath? What if you could not? That's what happens when your oxygen supply line (Zones 2 and 3) is blocked in your sleep by the tongue. Your conscious brain may be asleep, but not your autonomic nervous system in charge of your survival.

As your blood oxygen level drops, the survival director springs into rescue mission: "Code Blue! Start CPR! Mandible, move forward and pull the tongue with you out of the throat. Teeth are in the way? Get past them and fast! We are facing a life-or-death crisis. Get air in at all cost!"

Viewed from outside, this crisis mode typically involves snoring, leg kicking, chest heaving, and elbowing the sleep partner. The stress response inside may include high blood pressure, a pounding pulse, low oxygen concentration in the blood (so the body is acidic and "turns blue"), teeth grinding, acid reflux that can dissolve tooth enamel, acute-stress hormones that irritate the bladder (interrupting sleep with bathroom calls), and difficulty going back to sleep. All the while, a tissue rusting process called oxidative stress is aging the body rather than refreshing it with deep sleep.

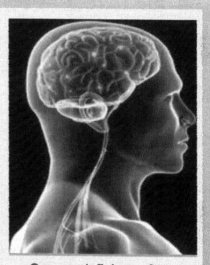

Teeth Grinders Often Suffer These Symptoms:

* Dental sensitivities
* Gum recession, broken teeth
* Sore jaws, clicking jaw joints
* Bladder urgency
* Morning headaches
* Daytime sleepiness
* Body Aches and pains
* Brain fog, poor memory
* Depression, moodiness
* Chronic fatigue, adrenal exhaustion
* High blood pressure
* Higher dental and medical bills

Oxygen deficiency from airway obstruction is why.

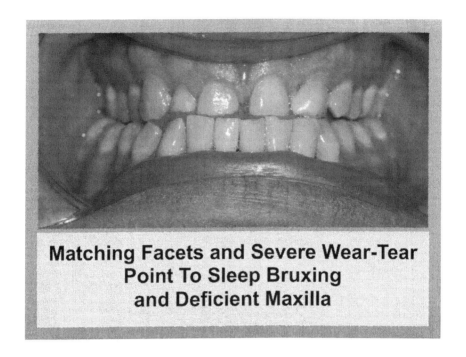

Matching Facets and Severe Wear-Tear Point To Sleep Bruxing and Deficient Maxilla

Sleep Bruxing Airway Disorder: Telling the Truth in Teeth Grinding

By now you know bruxing is not just a dental problem, which is why most night guards do not stop teeth grinding. A night guard does not rescue the airway, nor does it address the cause.

Based on the Code Blue inside story above, and the scientific evidence linking teeth grinding and sleep apnea below, I now see each night guard as a missed opportunity to help the patient both dentally and medically.

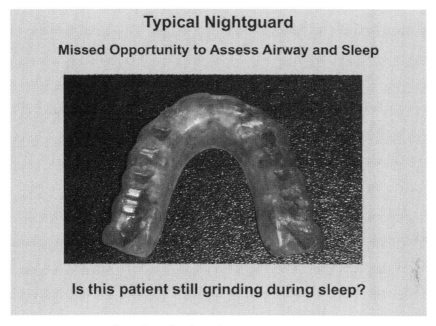

*The red marks show that this night guard is
registering teeth grinding, not stopping it.*

I propose that teeth grinding be seen as Sleep Bruxing Airway Disorder (SBAD) to truly reflect its origin and nature and therefore to direct its treatment at the anatomical source.

But before we look at the new way to address the cause, let's look into the science connecting sleep, airway, and mouth structure.

Teeth Grinding Is Widespread

General dentists I have polled informally say they see grinding in 50 to 80 percent of their patients. The more WholeHealth-minded the dentist, the more they see.

Studies on teeth-grinding prevalence vary widely, a likely result of studies relying on self-reporting because the patients are asleep when they brux (and, if a child, in a different room from their parent). For instance, one Stanford study that relied on self-reporting found that 8.2 percent of a large sample (over 11,000) admitted to bruxing. [3]

Yet a Brazilian study found that "bruxism occurs in nearly 60 percent of children between ages 3 and 5, with important repercussions." [4]

The criteria used may explain the big discrepancy in teeth grinding rate in the patient population. Patients/Parents understandably use sound, while dentists use matching wear facets on opposing teeth. Bite your teeth firmly together and rub them side-to-side and front-and-back. There is likely no sound. Repeat the same while looking into the mirror, and you will likely see matching wear facts.

Other studies have cast light on the relationship between sleep apnea and bruxing. For instance, research out of Baylor College of Medicine found that 25% of sleep apnea patients were also bruxers. [5]

Another study, this out of the University of British Columbia in Vancouver, found that 54% of mild and 40% of moderate sleep apnea patients also bruxed. "It appears," wrote the authors, "that sleep bruxism is…related to the disturbed sleep of OSA patients." [6]

The Link Between Teeth Grinding and Sleep Apnea

According to a 2007 Canadian study, bruxing is related to the stress activation of the heart and brain during sleep. [7] The mouth is part of coordinated "multi-media" response to the life-threatening stress of oxygen deprivation from airway obstruction.

So, what might activate stress during sleep? I propose that the real perpetrator is the "three-foot cage" — a structurally impaired mouth with jaws too small to house a normal-sized tongue, thereby forcing it into the throat space reserved for oxygen delivery.

An Impaired Mouth thus drives the tongue to clog the airway, which results in teeth grinding on the dental side and obstructive sleep apnea (OSA) on the medical side. In fact, OSA is the highest risk factor for bruxism. [8] Both are associated with high blood pressure, acid reflux, chronic pain, and many other systemic symptoms. [9, 10, 11, 12]

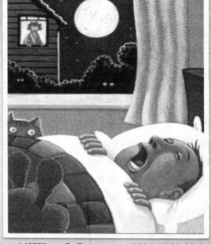

Obstructive Sleep Apnea (OSA) Symptoms:

- High blood pressure, stroke*
- Heart attack, sudden death*
- Diabetes, obesity*
- GERD: acid reflux*
- Lower immunity*
- Depression, anxiety*
- Brain fog, senile memory*
- Accelerated aging*
- Chronic pain*
- Daytime sleepiness, accidents*
- Teeth Grinding (Dr. Liao's input)

* William C. Dement and Merrill M. Mitler, *JAMA* 269, no. 12 (1993): 1548–1550.

Seeing teeth grinding as an early warning of airway struggle can, in my opinion, prevent subsequent heart disease, brain degeneration, chronic pain, feature, and mood problems.

Sleep bruxing is an unconscious reaction to oxygen deprivation with the collapse of zones 2 and 3 (see image below). Treating the deficient maxilla and mandible as needed to widen that "three-foot cage" as part of a overall wellness program can help reverse the symptoms naturally.

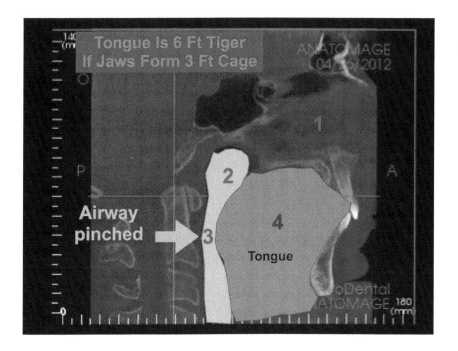

Teeth grinding is defined as "a repetitive jaw-muscle activity characterized by clenching or grinding of the teeth and/or by bracing or thrusting of the mandible." [13] Sleep bruxing is classified as a sleep-related movement disorder by the American Academy of Sleep Medicine. [14]

Now you can understand why teeth grinding is called sleep bruxing — to highlight its connection with sleep.

Dental Complications of Teeth Grinding

Dentally, teeth grinding is diagnosed from matching wear facets on opposing teeth and a gradual shortening of teeth. Most patients are not aware that they grind since it occurs when the conscious brain is off-duty. Some grinders may feel soreness or stiffness around their ears, temples, and cheeks, and feel unrefreshed when they wake up. Others may not – at least until they wind up at the dentist's office with bruxing complications, which can and often include:

- Loss of natural teeth and compromised smile attractiveness.

- Gum recession and gaps between teeth.

- Sensitive teeth and loosened teeth.

- Broken teeth, loosened crowns, and dead nerves in well-brushed and flossed teeth.

- Dental nerve inflammation requiring root-canals after dental work.

- Persistent pain and nagging discomfort after root-canal treatment.

- Cracked teeth necessitating extractions and expensive bridgework.

- Bone loss around natural teeth roots and failing dental implants.

- Clicking, popping, and locking jaw joints.

- Pain in the jaws, face, head, neck, shoulders and back, fatigue, depression, anxiety, anger, unexplained hostility, and other systemic symptoms.

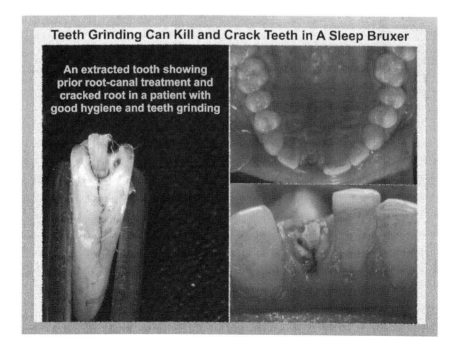

Teeth Grinding Can Kill and Crack Teeth in A Sleep Bruxer

An extracted tooth showing prior root-canal treatment and cracked root in a patient with good hygiene and teeth grinding

The image below shows the mouth of a patient with straight white teeth, generalized gum recession (yellow arrows), midline discrepancy of her upper and lower front teeth, and matching wear facets. She experienced chronic fatigue, frequent colds, and Lyme disease for years. The common thread among all her symptoms is chronic oxygen deficiency from airway obstruction during sleep.

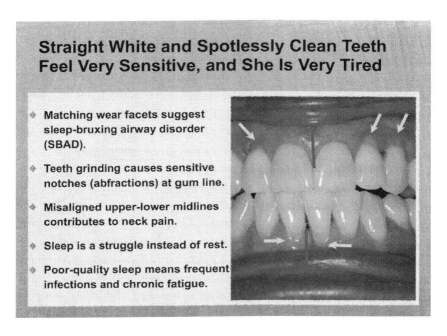

Straight White and Spotlessly Clean Teeth Feel Very Sensitive, and She Is Very Tired

- Matching wear facets suggest sleep-bruxing airway disorder (SBAD).
- Teeth grinding causes sensitive notches (abfractions) at gum line.
- Misaligned upper-lower midlines contributes to neck pain.
- Sleep is a struggle instead of rest.
- Poor-quality sleep means frequent infections and chronic fatigue.

In my experience, patients with persistent Lyme symptoms often have deficient airway and Impaired Mouth. This can make a great research study.

While you often hear that stress causes teeth grinding, "psychiatric or psychological factors do not play a role in most cases," according to the National Sleep Foundation. Oxygen deprivation from the tongue obstructing the airway is a greater threat to survival than psychological stress.

"Use of certain medications, including amphetamines, are… associated with episodes of bruxism." [15] If you are on anti-depressants or psychiatric medications, check for their side effects and discuss with your doctor.

In my experience, stress dissipates and mood lifts when sleep normalizes, and teeth grinding stops once the airway is unblocked.

Jaws Muscles and Sleep Studies

Before we go any further, it will be helpful to get to get acquainted with a couple of your jaw muscles, which can matter in toothaches and teeth grinding.

Put the palms of your hands on your cheeks, with the webs of your thumbs around your earlobes and the tips of your fingers over your temples. Clench your jaws and grind your teeth. Do you feel the jaw muscles bulge under your hands? The *masseter* muscles are the big chewing muscles against your palms, while the *temporalis* muscles are the ones under your fingers.

Trigger points are taut bands or painful knots in muscles. What makes them trigger points is that their pain actually arises from a different source. Their identification was a significant contribution to medical science by Drs. Janet Travell and David Simons [16].

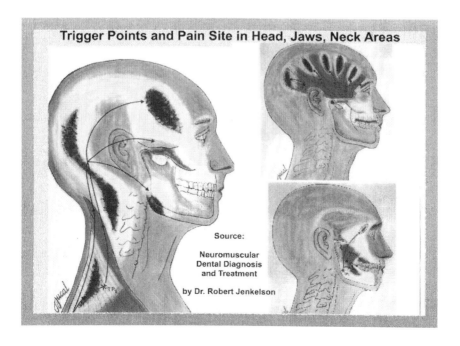

Trigger Points and Pain Site in Head, Jaws, Neck Areas

Source:

Neuromuscular
Dental Diagnosis
and Treatment

by Dr. Robert Jenkelson

In the head and neck region, trigger points are often found on the top of the shoulders (the *trapezius* muscle), on the sides of the neck (the *sternocleidomastoid, or SCM*), and in jaw muscles such as the temporalis and masseter.

Trigger points in the trapezius and SCM can bring on aches and pains in the jaws, ears, sinuses, and teeth, especially if pain persists after root-canal treatment — see chapters 8 and 11.

The masseter and temporalis are the surface muscles of your masticatory (chewing) apparatus, and their activities can be recorded as electrical readouts using electromyography (EMG), which is included in sleep tests. Sleep bruxism shows up on EMG characteristically as "repetitive and recurrent episodes of rhythmic masticatory muscle activity (RMMA) of the masseter and temporalis muscles that are usually associated with sleep arousals." [17]

This means jaw clenching and teeth grinding can interrupt sleep without your awareness. "Clenching and grinding is actually an attempt to protect the airway," says Dr. Jerald H. Simmons, a neurologist and sleep disorder specialist in Houston. [18] That's because when those chewing muscles are activated, the throat relaxes to make swallowing possible.

Teeth grinding is one way to move the tongue out of the airway while the body tries to stay asleep, in my view.

Sleep Bruxing: A Brain-Mediated Stress Event

Sleep bruxing sacrifices teeth for a higher cause — to resuscitate the whole body in times of airway obstruction during sleep. Rather than some isolated dental event, it is a brain-mediated response to acute oxygen starvation. Here's the evidence:

- Deep sleep goes shallower 10 seconds before teeth grinding, and the heart rate goes up around the start of grinding, according to a 1997 study from Sweden's University of

Gothenburg. Bruxing was also associated with micro-arousals and stress during sleep. [19]

Teeth Grinding = Sleep Bruxing = Micro-Arousals in Brain During Sleep

Source: Gaby G. Bader and others, *SLEEP* 20, no. 11 (1997): 982–990.

- Micro-arousals of 3-15" in REM + light sleep.
- EEG spikes 4" before bruxing event.
- Heart rate spikes 10" after = stress.
- Oxygen deficit => sympathetic nervous system activation.
- Jaw movement + chest + limbs.
- Teeth grinding may be an oral manifestation of airway obstruction during sleep.

Abfractions: suspect teeth grinding.

- Here's why grinding can leave you feeling tired when you wake up: a 2007 study from the University of Montreal confirmed the findings of the Sweden study, showing that stress events come before chewing muscle activation in sleep bruxing. The researchers noted that 86% of bruxism occurred "during periods of sleep arousal" and found that muscle activity was "3 times higher in patients with sleep bruxing than in controls, and is typically associated with tooth-grinding sounds (in 45 percent of cases), as reported by patients, bed partners, parents, or siblings. [20]

- However, not all RMMA episodes are accompanied by tooth grinding, and many patients or family members may not be aware of this." [20]

- Blood pressure surges 20 to 25 percent after teeth-grinding events, reports a 2012 study in SLEEP. [21] This is worth knowing if you have high blood pressure.

- "Taken all evidence together," write the authors of a 2001 paper, "bruxism appears to be mainly regulated centrally, not peripherally." [22] This means teeth grinding is a brain-mediated stress response and thus cannot be fixed inside the dental box.

On computed tomography (CT) imaging, chronic jaw muscle contractions appear as bony outgrowths at the angle of the lower jaw. See the arrows on the image below. This is a useful diagnostic feature in connecting teeth grinding to sleep apnea.

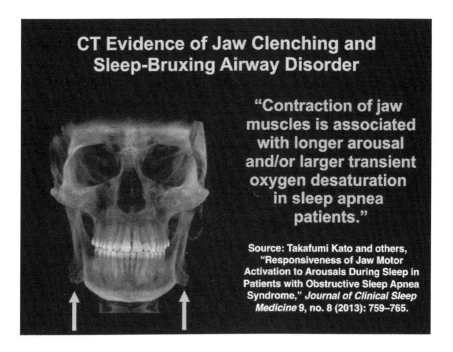

CT Evidence of Jaw Clenching and Sleep-Bruxing Airway Disorder

"Contraction of jaw muscles is associated with longer arousal and/or larger transient oxygen desaturation in sleep apnea patients."

Source: Takafumi Kato and others, "Responsiveness of Jaw Motor Activation to Arousals During Sleep in Patients with Obstructive Sleep Apnea Syndrome," *Journal of Clinical Sleep Medicine* 9, no. 8 (2013): 759–765.

Suggested Clinical Management of Sleep Bruxing

So, what can be done about teeth grinding? Here is what one review article on sleep bruxing suggests:

- To control and prevent tooth wear, an intraoral appliance is recommended.

- However, because the patient is already a snorer and presents anatomic risk factors for SDB [sleep disordered breathing], an MAA [mandibular advancement appliance] would be preferable to an occlusal or stabilization splint [night guard].

- Follow-up visits must be scheduled to customize and adjust the MAA, verify the patient's general and oral status (stress level), and prevent sleep-bruxing consequences (tooth wear, pain) from worsening. [23]

To the above, we can now add a new a new type of oral appliance, targeting both the upper and lower jaws, the mandible and maxilla alike. Now let's take a look at a real-life case next using Impaired Mouth diagnosis and Holistic Mouth as a natural solution.

Holistic Mouth Nuggets

- Teeth grinding (sleep bruxing) is a sign of airway obstruction and a brain-mediated response to the threat to survival from oxygen deficiency during sleep. It is the price of trying to move the tongue out of the airway while the body tries to stay asleep.

- Sleep bruxing disrupts sleep and robs rest, bodily repair, and energy regeneration. It is a reaction to choked airway that accelerates adrenal exhaustion, degeneration, and aging.

- Seeing teeth grinding as Sleep Bruxing Airway Disorder (SBAD) points to its true origin and directs its treatment at the anatomical source.

- Seeing teeth grinding is an early warning of airway struggle can lead to treatment for preventing or reversing subsequent heart disease, brain degeneration, chronic pain, feature, and mood problems.

Chapter 5

"I Ground Through My Night Guard" — A Holistic Mouth Solutions Case Study

I am constantly amazed at how powerful a predictor of health your teeth are.

– Dr. Joseph Mercola [1]

"I'm here because I had ground through my night guard," said R.H., a young woman who had been referred to me by her mom's orthogonal chiropractic doctor who specializes in aligning the head squarely over the top of the neck. As an aspiring tennis player, R.H. was interested in having more energy. As R.H.'s biggest fan, her mom was interested in more victories and superior health for R.H.

R.H. was a severe teeth grinder. She wore a night guard, but judging from the wear, it didn't appear to have done much good. At the age of 17, her teeth showed the wear and tear of a 71-year old.

Although she had finished orthodontics three years earlier, R.H. also had an anterior (front of the mouth) open bite. It came from tongue thrust – more evidence that her tongue's habitat was just too small.

"You have an intelligent tongue," I told her. "It doesn't want to be occupying your very narrow airway."

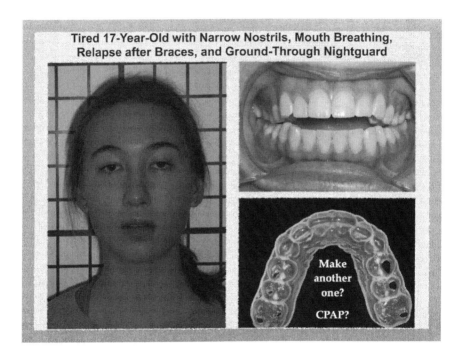

Tired 17-Year-Old with Narrow Nostrils, Mouth Breathing, Relapse after Braces, and Ground-Through Nightguard

Make another one?

CPAP?

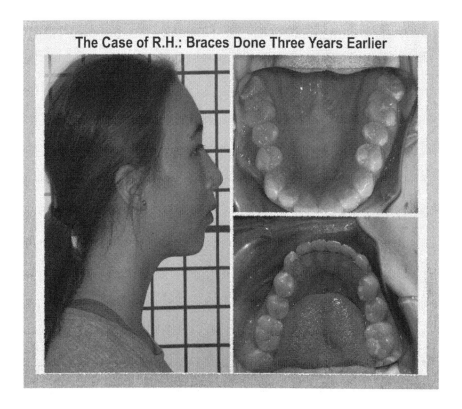

The Case of R.H.: Braces Done Three Years Earlier

I asked R.H. and her mom if they wanted another night guard, or if they would rather help lead the "tiger" out of her airway by redeveloping her deficient maxilla. They chose to take a new path.

CSI: Clues of an Impaired Mouth

While the bruxing and anterior bite were clear signs of an impaired mouth and pinched airway, baseline records and cephalometric analysis showed even more clues:

- Facially, R.H. looked tired, and the whites under the irises of the eyes were visible, which indicates an underdeveloped maxilla. [2]

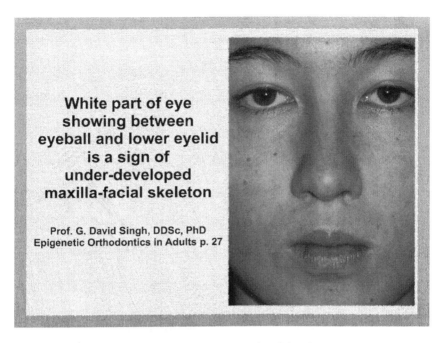

White part of eye showing between eyeball and lower eyelid is a sign of under-developed maxilla-facial skeleton

Prof. G. David Singh, DDSc, PhD
Epigenetic Orthodontics in Adults p. 27

- R.H. had a forward head posture in side view and a head tilt in frontal view. She had habitual mouth breathing, constricted nostrils, and chapped lips.

- Dentally, R.H. had severe wear of the posterior (back) teeth, which indicated bruxing and suggested airway obstruction. Because of her tongue thrust, her front teeth were "bucked" forward by more than 10 degrees compared with the normal range. Her narrow jaws and high palatal vault indicated an underdeveloped maxilla. Her tongue position blocked the view of her uvula, suggesting a high risk of sleep apnea. [3]

- CT imaging showed that her airway diameter was 3 mm, about 25 percent of low normal. Her airway volume was 7.7 cc, less than half of low normal (20 cc). Cephalometric analysis revealed that her maxilla was retruded by 8 mm, and her mandible was retruded by 12 mm relative to her head. This left her tongue no choice but to occupy her airway.

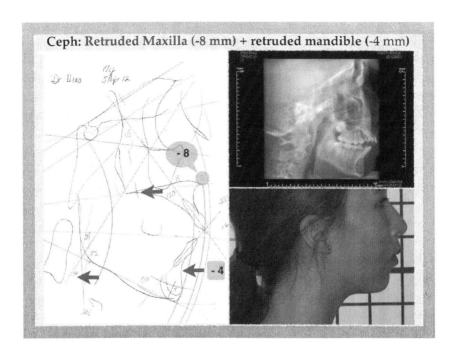

Ceph: Retruded Maxilla (-8 mm) + retruded mandible (-4 mm)

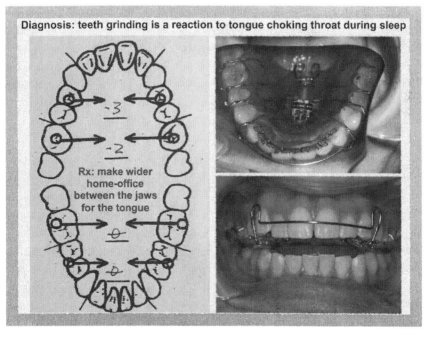

Diagnosis: teeth grinding is a reaction to tongue choking throat during sleep

Rx: make wider home-office between the jaws for the tongue

R.H.'s tongue did not want to be stuck in her throat. So, it fought its way out by forcing open the front end of its "cage." The tongue has the power to shape the jaws and the face.

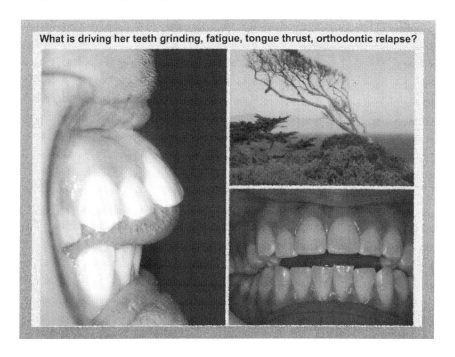

What is driving her teeth grinding, fatigue, tongue thrust, orthodontic relapse?

A Holistic Mouth Solution for R.H.

With all this evidence in hand, I developed a treatment plan to re-form R.H.'s "three-foot cage" as follows:

- Wear an upper arch biomimetic oral appliance – the DNA appliance – for 16 hours a day, from sunset to breakfast. Widen is by 0.25 mm twice a week.

- Wear an oral face mask ("headgear") attached to her appliance from after dinner until breakfast the next morning to gently pull the maxilla forward during sleep.

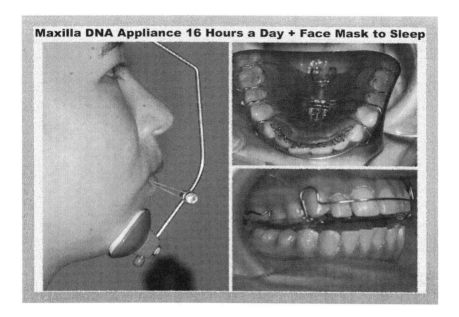

Maxilla DNA Appliance 16 Hours a Day + Face Mask to Sleep

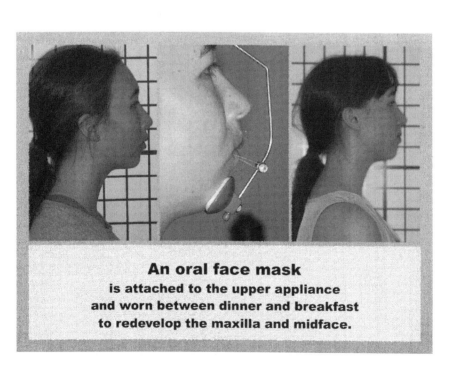

An oral face mask
is attached to the upper appliance
and worn between dinner and breakfast
to redevelop the maxilla and midface.

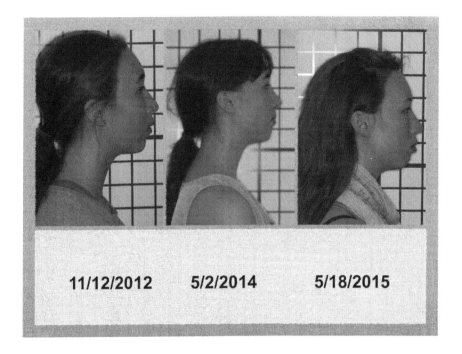

11/12/2012   5/2/2014   5/18/2015

- Improve her sleep hygiene: to sleep by 11pm, blackout blinds in the bedroom, no LED lights or cellphones in the bedroom after 11 pm.
- Eat organic foods and follow the Nourishing Traditions diet [4] to promote bone growth and healthy development.
- See and orthogonal chiropractic doctor as needed.
- Do orofacial myofunctional and Buteyko breathing exercises to turn habitual mouth breathing into full-time nose breathing. [5, 6, 7]

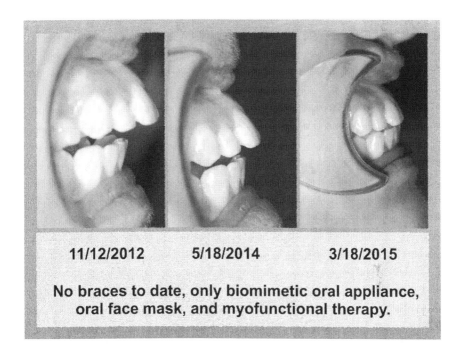

11/12/2012   5/18/2014   3/18/2015

No braces to date, only biomimetic oral appliance,
oral face mask, and myofunctional therapy.

A Wider Airway and No More Bruxing

To her credit, R.H. did do her part, and faithfully. After 10 months of oral appliance therapy, R.H. reported the happy results:

> I came to Dr. Liao looking for a new night guard — I had ground holes in it. I had been losing my tennis matches (I am a tennis player) and did not know why. Dr. Liao made me realize that my airway was 75 percent blocked and my tongue was too big for my mouth. Doing oral appliance therapy for 10 months has changed my whole life: I don't grind my teeth anymore, my whole profile has changed, I am sleeping better, and I am winning my matches now. Best of all, the whites under my eyes are gone."

Over eighteen months of therapy, R.H's airway volume more than tripled, increasing from 7.7 cc to 24 cc. This gave her all the oxygen her body needed to flower into her full genetic potential. [8]

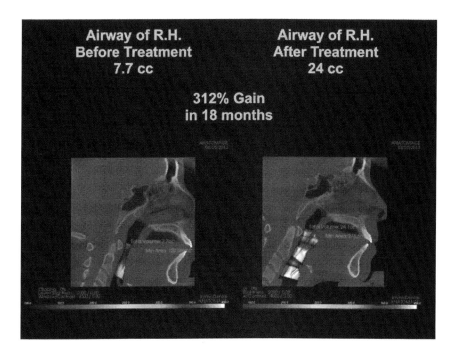

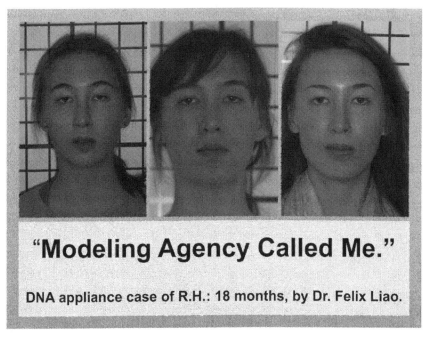

Different Outcome Requires Different Thinking

Treating airway obstruction stops teeth grinding, sleep apnea, and their related complications. Would R.H. have ground through her second and third night guards if she had stayed inside the traditional dental silo?

By choosing oral appliance therapy over a night guard, R.H. saved herself many medical and dental woes down the road, not to mention health care costs. That is the first lesson her case teaches.

Secondly, it affirms that oral appliance therapy cannot be successful without patient effort. R.H. and her parents deserve credit for contributing to the positive result with their 100% compliance. R.H. wore the appliance as directed and followed the prescribed Holistic Mouth treatment faithfully, and she did her myofunctional therapy homework to increase her lip strength and tone and retrain her tongue posture.

Healthier use of the mouth is just important as oral appliance therapy. R.H. switched from the typical American junk diet to organic whenever possible. For while oral appliance therapy – correctly diagnosed and designed – can help jumpstart health recovery and improve sleep, it cannot overcome the misuse, abuse, and overuse of the mouth with junk food, sugary drinks, excessive carbs, caffeine, alcohol, dairy, and so on. Patients are referred for nutritional coaching whenever indicated, but R.H. did it herself. I only had to give advice once.

Would R.H.'s outcome have been possible without her active, positive participation? No. Could her epigenetic orthopedic oral appliance fix her habitual mouth breathing and standard American eating habits? No.

It is the teamwork of the patient as her/his mouth's owner-operator AND a Holistic Mouth doctor with the necessary WholeHealth knowledge to connect the necessary dots and carry out a treatment plan that lets the body respond favorably.

This is how Holistic Mouth Solutions™ actualize genetic potential for beautiful and happy outcome.

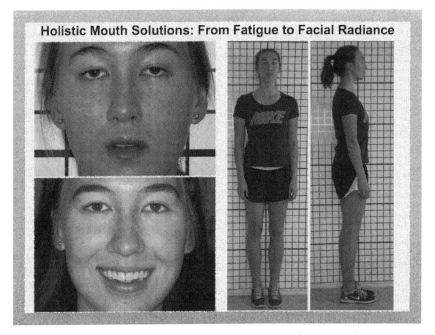

Holistic Mouth Solutions: From Fatigue to Facial Radiance

*Radiant health four years after starting Holistic Mouth
Solutions, without needing another night guard.*

R.H. came back to see me two years later for a check-up and cleaning. She brought a boyfriend with her. When I asked why it had been so long since I had seen her, she said, "I've just been too busy playing and teaching tennis, modeling, and having a great time!"

Life can be great with a Holistic Mouth supporting whole body health through ABCDES: alignment breathing circulation, digestion, energy, and sleep. I have no doubt that R.H. will enjoy all of that throughout her life.

Holistic Mouth Nuggets

- Treating teeth grinding with night guards misses the opportunity to investigate airway distress and possibly intercept sleep apnea early on. R.H.'s case shows fuller genetic potential can show up when the airway is treated as a cause of teeth grinding.

- Recognition of teeth grinding as a sleep bruxing airway disorder (SBAD) an opportunity to turn oral and systemic health toward fuller genetic potential.

- Oral appliances do not by themselves fix patients' problems by themselves. It takes close collaboration between a compliant patient and a doctor of Holistic Mouth to translate epigenetic orthopedics and WholeHealth principles into a happy and beautiful outcome.

Chapter 5

Holistic Mouth Epigenetics — Harnessing Your Stem Cells to Put Your Best Face Forward

Facial and body disproportions/abnormalities are due to environmental factors and significantly less to genetics.

– Dr. Yosh Jefferson [1]

R.H.'s face changed naturally and her airway volume tripled after her oral appliance therapy, yet she had the same genes throughout. So, what explains her facial transformation? The answer starts with those stem cells in the sockets of healthy teeth, and a new type of treatment called *epigenetic orthopedics*. Let's unpack these big new words.

Epigenetic Orthopedics

Two-thirds of the face is framed by the jaws – the upper, called the *maxilla*, and the lower, called the *mandible*. The face you now have is the combination of your genes and your epigenetics.

Epi- means "on top of" or "in addition to." And "epigenetics" are factors that influence how your genes express themselves. Habitual mouth breathing is one example of an epigenetic influence on facial development. Diet and exercise are also epigenetics. A figure skater who grew up skating has a very different form than if she had simply sat and played video games.

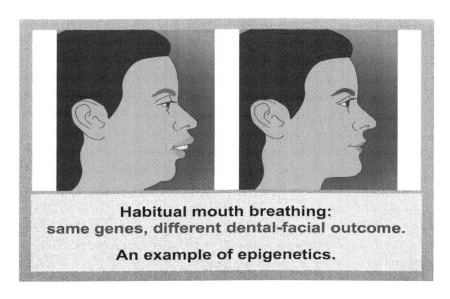

Habitual mouth breathing: same genes, different dental-facial outcome.

An example of epigenetics.

Ortho- is Greek for straight, right-angled, or correct. Orthopedic medicine began as a correction of skeletal deformities in children. In the craniofacial context, *orthopedics* involves bone-to-bone relationship of how maxilla-mandible relationships, while *orthodontics* refers to teeth-to-teeth relationships.

Epigenetic craniofacial orthopedics, then, is the redevelopment of an impaired mouth, addressing jaw size, position, and dental occlusion (bite) using Holistic Mouth Solutions. Thanks in part to the work of Dr. G. Dave Singh, a pioneer in epigenetic jaw and airway redevelopment, we can now make these changes in adults – something thought to be impossible until recent advances in epigenetics. The benefits are many, including better nasal breathing and sinus drainage, less anxiety, higher cheek bones, fuller lips, natural facial radiance, and more.

Age is Not a Factor: C.S.'s Story

C.S. was 66 years old when she began her epigenetic oral orthopedic appliance therapy. Five months in, she reported the improvements:

> After about the first ten days, I started sleeping through the night and dreaming for the first time in years. My posture and my gait is much better — the oral appliance took away my knee pain I had lived with for the past ten years. I am totally pleased with it.

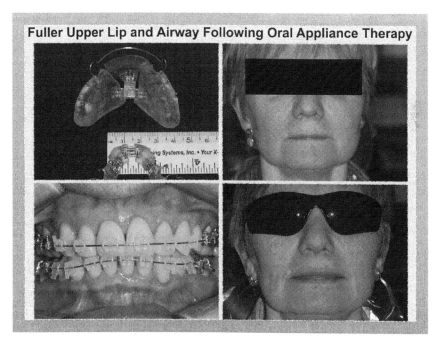

Note the change in C.S.'S lips after oral appliance therapy — closer to her genetic potential.

To be clear, the appliance did not do all the work. C.S.'s Holistic Mouth Solutions included myofunctional therapy, nasal breathing exercises, postural training, acupuncture treatment, and a bone-building diet. Her case shows what can happen to total health when the tongue gets a suitable habitat between the jaws, and when the patient is fully compliant.

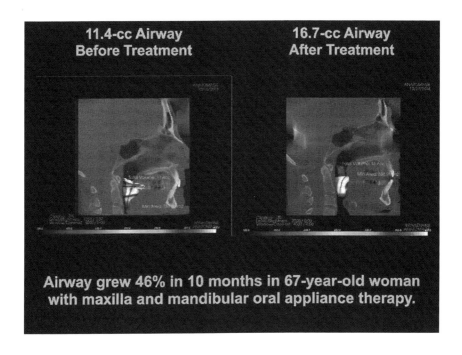

11.4-cc Airway Before Treatment · **16.7-cc Airway After Treatment**

Airway grew 46% in 10 months in 67-year-old woman with maxilla and mandibular oral appliance therapy.

This case also drives home the point that epigenetic orthopedic redevelopment works regardless of age, as long as the patient (A) is willing to do the required "homework", and (B) has enough good teeth in sound bone.

"I am too old" from the patient is no longer an excuse, and "You are too old" from the doctor is no longer valid.

Epigenetics: Telling Your Genes What to Do

Genes are biological codes for making proteins that give form to your body and face. They contain the molecular blueprints you are born with. Growth starts when genes are turned on and stops when genes are turned off. Epigenetic orthopedic appliances signal the genes and tell them to resume growing the jaws as if the patient is undergoing teenage growth spurt.

Epigenetic factors shape *what* you end up with. A child with habitual mouth breathing and enlarged tonsils, for instance, can grow up with a less attractive adult face. As Dr. Yosh Jefferson notes in a paper for *General Dentistry*, "Children whose mouth breathing is untreated may develop long, narrow faces, narrow mouths, high palatal vaults, dental malocclusion, gummy smiles, and many other unattractive facial features, such as skeletal Class II or Class III (less optimal than Class I) facial profiles. These children do not sleep well at night due to obstructed airways; this lack of sleep can adversely affect their growth and academic performance. Many of these children are misdiagnosed with attention deficit disorder (ADD) and hyperactivity." [3]

This is why a Holistic Mouth doctor pays attention to nasal airway and works with integrative health professionals to ensure that the nose is functionally unobstructed and structurally wide enough.

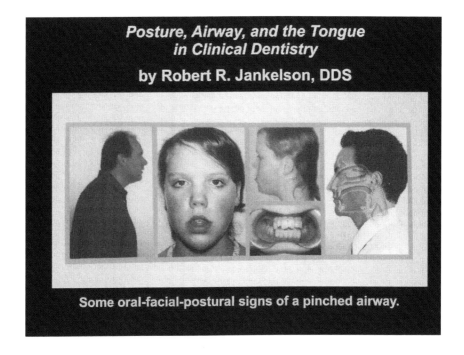

Posture, Airway, and the Tongue in Clinical Dentistry
by Robert R. Jankelson, DDS

Some oral-facial-postural signs of a pinched airway.

Epigenetic factors tell your genes what to do, where to do it, and when. These factors can be from natural sources like food or from human-made sources like medicines or pesticides, according to the National Human Genome Research Institute. [4] Where stem cells are available, oral appliances can serve as an epigenetic stimulus, as well, triggering genes to resume development toward their full potential in the oral-facial region.

But just what *is* "full genetic potential"?

Craniofacial Development: Full Genetic Potential

Scientifically speaking, the *craniofacial skeleton* consists of the 22 bones that make up the head: 8 for the cranium and 14 for the face. It changes in size, shape, and complexity from no teeth at birth to 24 teeth at age 7, to 32 teeth around age 18. Along the way, teeth can end up naturally straight in good *occlusion* (bite) or in *malocclusion* (bad bite).

With good genes and favorable epigenetics, the mouth can become a health asset (a Holistic Mouth) and the face can look radiant from good sleep night after night. With good genes and bad epigenetics, the mouth can develop into a health liability (an impaired mouth), and the face can look downcast.

Development is the change in physical size, shape, and complexity over time based on the genes. Underdevelopment happens when growth is turned off prematurely by epigenetic factors. Underdevelopment results in an impaired mouth with poor form, inferior function, and more health problems. Common signs of impaired mouth include various combinations of crowded teeth, weak chin, flat cheekbones, sunken midface, clicking jaw joints, and all the medical-dental-mood complications of snoring, sleep apnea, and teeth grinding.

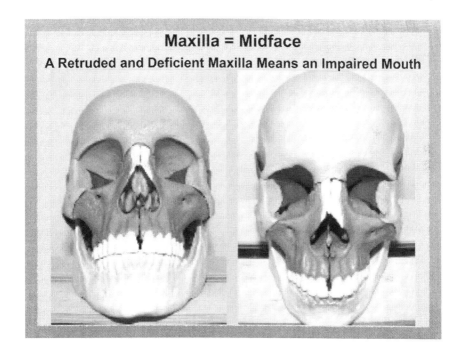

81

Holistic Mouth Means Reaching Full Genetic Potential

Full genetic potential in craniofacial development is reached when the two jaws have enough room for all 32 teeth without crowding and enough oral volume for the tongue to stay in the mouth, i.e. out of the airway, day and night. That's what a Holistic Mouth represents — fuller genetic potential.

Some excellent examples of full genetic potential come from the indigenous populations studied by Dr. Weston A. Price. [5] Without toothbrushes, dental floss, pediatricians, orthodontists, supplements, or health insurance, these humans managed to grow up with wide jaws, naturally straight teeth, few or no cavities, and radiant natural health.

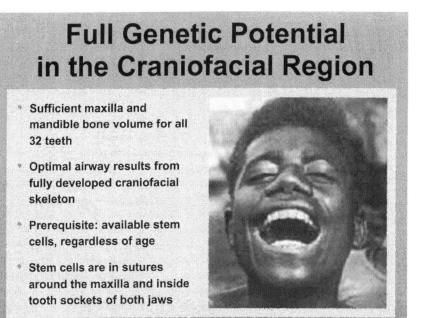

Full Genetic Potential in the Craniofacial Region

* Sufficient maxilla and mandible bone volume for all 32 teeth

* Optimal airway results from fully developed craniofacial skeleton

* Prerequisite: available stem cells, regardless of age

* Stem cells are in sutures around the maxilla and inside tooth sockets of both jaws

Human take 15 to 20 years to mature into adult form, which is a long time for epigenetic forces to drive jaw development off course. The cumulative burdens of modern living, processed foods, and increased mouth breathing from allergies all contribute to today's higher incidence of malocclusion, facial imbalance, impaired mouths, and pinched airways. In contrast, the radiant faces and wide arches with naturally straight teeth in these individuals can serve as "true north" for patients, parents, dentists, and all health professionals.

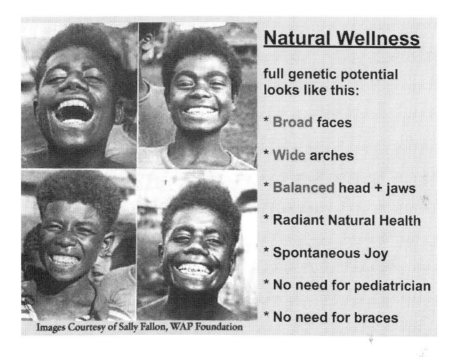

Natural Wellness

full genetic potential looks like this:

* Broad faces

* Wide arches

* Balanced head + jaws

* Radiant Natural Health

* Spontaneous Joy

* No need for pediatrician

* No need for braces

Images Courtesy of Sally Fallon, WAP Foundation

Nutrition is an especially important epigenetic factor as documented by Dr. Price. In photographs like the ones below, you can see what he identified as the consequences of a "modern" diet, with its refined sugar, white flour, and other highly processed foods. In addition to the loss of teeth to cavities, the next generation showed longer, narrower faces, and malocclusion was evident.

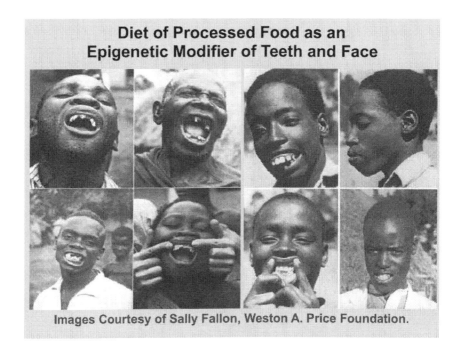

Diet of Processed Food as an Epigenetic Modifier of Teeth and Face

Images Courtesy of Sally Fallon, Weston A. Price Foundation.

Dr. Price's findings were later confirmed by Dr. Francis Pottenger's study of cats: "If proper nutrition and exercise are absent when facial structures are developing, dentition always suffers. The kitten kept on a deficient diet for 10 months has an inadequate jaw with crowded, irregular, and poorly aligned teeth." [6]

Epigenetic Factors and Science

How you live, eat, drink, and sleep can stunt or promote growth and development — that's what epigenetics says. "The epigenome is made up of chemical compounds and proteins that can attach to DNA and direct such actions as turning genes on or off, controlling the production of proteins in particular cells." [7]

In my experience, epigenetic factors that can interfere with craniofacial development include malnutrition, physical/emotional distress, illness, exposure to toxins during pregnancy, unhealthy family dynamics (alcohol, drug, or physical abuse), maternal pelvic asymmetry, birth trauma to the newborn's cranial (skull) bones, tongue-tie, bottle feeding, improper weaning, overuse of pacifier, habitual mouth breathing, tongue thrusting, thumb sucking, processed foods that favor inflammation (high sugar) or degeneration (pesticides, preservatives), and excessive antibiotics resulting in dysbiosis (bad bacteria dominating over good bacteria).

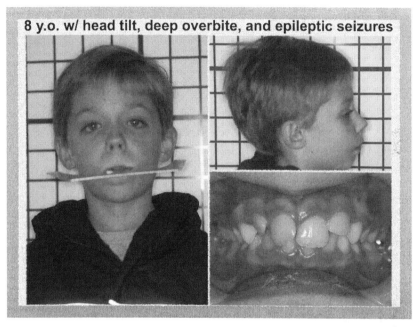

This 8 year-old boy's granmal epileptic seizures stopped after the correction of his deep overbite and nutritional support of adding sea food and marine vegetables and eggs to his diet — see chapter 18 for a slideshow of his progress.

Epigenetic factors that promote full genetic expressions can include maternal nutrition (folate, minerals, and fat-soluble vitamins A, D, and E) and the expectant mom's craniofacial-spinal-pelvic alignment, love, security, a non-traumatic birth process, breast feeding, proper weaning, full time nasal breathing with lip seal, and bone-building nutrition such as the Nourishing Traditions diet during the growth years. [8]

Epigenetic factors can also include corrective treatment modalities such as epigenetic orthopedic oral appliances, myofunctional therapy, tongue-tie release, nasal breathing full-time to correct habitual mouth breathing [9], a healthy lifestyle with sleep hygiene in sync with circadian rhythms, ensuring digestive health and hormonal balance, and stress management.

Unfortunately, deviated dental-facial-postural development is increasingly the rule rather than exception, in my experience. Given the serious consequences on total health from an impaired mouth on individual health and our national treasury, an understanding of epigenetic orthopedics and its redevelopment is essential.

You Are No Longer Stuck with Impaired Mouth

As long as you have enough sound teeth and good bone, you are no longer stuck with an impaired mouth all your life. Craniofacial epigenetics sees to that.

"Genes…do not function in isolation," says Dr. G. Dave Singh, a giant among my mentors. "Rather, they pick up developmental clues from the environment, leading to gene-environmental interaction, a phenomenon that can be summarized by the term 'epigenetics.'" [10] "In effect," Dr. Singh adds, "we can alter the phenotype (face) without altering the genotype (the genes) by expressing the unexpressed genes."

Translated: Impaired Mouth means stunted development, which can now be restarted with epigenetic oral appliances.

Epigenetics also says that pre- and post-natal nutrition is a factor that can affect cartilage formation and facial bone development. A 2015 Canadian study found that disturbance in cartilage growth "will produce coordinated shape changes in the adult calvarium [floor of the brain case] and face…. Strong reduction in cartilage growth produces a short, wide, and more flexed cranial base. This in turn produces a short, wide face … [in rats]." [11]

"Epigenetic changes can help determine whether genes are turned on or off," according to the National Library of Medicine. [12] This means you are not stuck with your impaired mouth and pinched airway, which amount to incomplete development that falls short of full genetic potential.

Conclusion: epigenetic orthopedic (biomimetic) appliances can signal the genetic assembly line to turn back on to make jaw bone according to your own genetic blueprint regardless of age.

Holistic Mouth Solutions™ to Actualize Fuller Genetic Potential

Holistic Mouth Solutions™ is a WholeHealth-oriented and customized treatment plan that includes nose breathing, functional lip and tongue pressure, and biomimetic appliances to signal the genes to resume bone development in the mid-face as if an adult were a teenager again.

Craniofacial epigenetics uses biomimetic appliances to stimulate the stem cells in and around the mouth to redevelop toward its full genetic potential. Genetic potential is "the optimal phenotypic (structural) outcome in the prevailing (environmental) conditions, subject to a viable population of stem cells." According to Professor G. Dave Singh, "Craniofacial epigenetics uses a person's natural genes to correct and straighten bones, soft tissues, teeth, and functional spaces painlessly using biomimetic appliances." [13]

And what does full genetic potential look like in the craniofacial region?

- Both the maxilla and the mandible are in proper alignment within the craniofacial skeleton, neither retruded nor excessively protruded.
- All 16 lower teeth line up straight within the mandible and maxilla, respectively.
- All upper and lower posterior teeth fit "peak-to-valley" in a stable and harmonious dental bite.
- The jaw joints can open and close in a straight path past 48 mm between upper and lower front teeth, and they pass the

"pinkie test." (Put your pinky fingers in your ear openings, with the finger pads facing forward. Feel for the jaw joints pushing against your finger pads when you bite, and listen for clicking, popping, or grating sounds. Such sounds suggest entrapment of the lower jaw and a tongue that is pinching the airway. Repeat the test but this time bite your front teeth together. This simulates the protruded position of the jaw joints. If the clicking noise and the pushback go away, then one or both jaws may be retruded.

- All orofacial soft tissues, including jaw muscles, tongue, lips, cheeks, and jaw joints are free of tension and pain, and free to reach full range of motion.

- The airway and nasal passage are wide enough to not interfere with deep, refreshing sleep.

With this understanding, let's look at a comparison of 2 brothers' cases.

Holistic Mouth Nuggets

- Genes determine what you are born with. Epigenetics shape what you end up with. Good genes + bad epigenetics = an impaired mouth and pinched airway.

- Good genes + good epigenetics = a Holistic Mouth and sufficient airway. A Holistic Mouth represents fully expressed genetic potential. An impaired mouth comes with pinched airway deficient jaws that can be redeveloped toward full genetic potential with epigenetic orthopedics.

- An epigenetic orthopedic (biomimetic) oral appliance can provide the epigenetic stimulus to "switch on" an individual's own genes to restart development toward a Holistic Mouth. This can work regardless of age, provided the patient has enough healthy teeth in sound bone – and does all the required "homework."

Chapter 6

Impaired Mouth Treated and Untreated — A Tale of Two Brothers' Cases

The International Diabetes Federation Taskforce on Epidemiology and Prevention strongly recommends that health professionals working in both type 2 diabetes and SDB [sleep-disordered breathing] adopt clinical practices to ensure that a patient presenting with one condition is considered for the other.

– Jonathan E. Shaw, et al [1]

This summary is worth repeating: Teeth grinding is not simply an dental event, but a brain-mediated stress reaction to "Code Blue" — oxygen deprivation from sleeping with a choked airway inside an Impaired Mouth.

As such, teeth grinding should be regarded as an early warning of sleep apnea risk ahead — long before the iceberg looms over the Titanic.

"Six-foot tiger, three-foot cage" states the problem AND suggests a solution. Can we offer a six-foot habitat for the tongue? If yes, will the snoring, bruxing, and daytime fatigue go away naturally? The answer to both questions is yes, but only if we expand our thinking beyond the night guard and the tooth-centered dental silo.

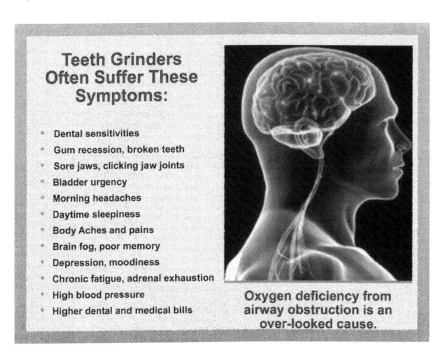

Teeth Grinders Often Suffer These Symptoms:

* Dental sensitivities
* Gum recession, broken teeth
* Sore jaws, clicking jaw joints
* Bladder urgency
* Morning headaches
* Daytime sleepiness
* Body Aches and pains
* Brain fog, poor memory
* Depression, moodiness
* Chronic fatigue, adrenal exhaustion
* High blood pressure
* Higher dental and medical bills

Oxygen deficiency from airway obstruction is an over-looked cause.

Pointing to the Cause and the Solution: Sleep Bruxing Airway Disorder

Whether you get to keep your teeth trouble-free for life depends not only on brushing, flossing, and eating well, but more critically a sufficient airway. A deficient airway inside an Impaired Mouth invariably result in excessive wear-and-tear from sleep bruxing with medical complications from sleep apnea. As I proposed in chapter 3, teeth grinding may be seen more accurately as *sleep bruxing airway disorder* (SBAD) to highlight airway obstruction as the anatomical cause of teeth grinding.

Teeth grinding is costly because you are born with a limited amount of enamel, that diamond-tough yet porcelain-smooth surface of teeth. Enamel makes natural teeth look white and beautiful, and is meant to outlast a lifetime. Pathological loss of enamel can come from cavities, excessive coarse or acidic foods (sucking on lemon), and/or teeth grinding. Enamel loss can result in exquisite sensitivity early on, and tens of thousands of dollars if sleep bruxing is left undetected and untreated.

Marie came to see me for a second opinion for a $90,000 dental reconstruction treatment plan which did not consider her sleep or airway. She had already spent upwards of $50,000 on her teeth before that because all 52 dentists she had seen in her lifetime just fixed one tooth after another.

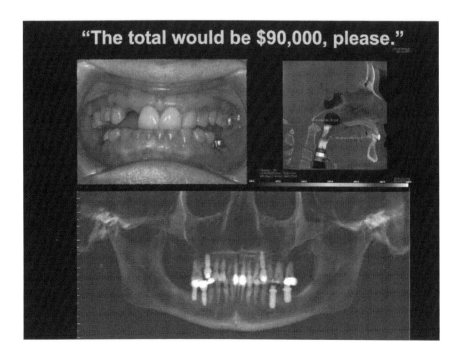

Given the degenerative nature of sleep apnea and the destructive outcome of bruxism, seeing teeth grinding as SBAD can better serve both dental patients with medical symptoms and dental patients with medical symptoms.

Given the widespread nature of both phenomena, dental health professionals trained to recognize Impaired Mouth can be a valuable resource for early screening and diagnostic referrals.

Seeing teeth grinding as SBAD makes all the difference for the patient in terms of treatment and outcome., as illustrated by the following cases of two brothers in their early 60s, both with sleep bruxing airway disorder.

The Case of A.K.

For over 30 years, A.K. would periodically travel across many state lines to see F.K., his brother and dentist. A.K. had had lots of dental problems, and his mouth was extremely difficult to work in because he could not open wide or long enough for dental work. He also had a strong gag reflex and an extremely "pushy" tongue that strongly defended its space. He had had an impacted upper canine that had lain inside his palate like a torpedo, the extraction of which had been a nightmare for him and his dentist brother.

Yet somehow, F.K. managed to get A.K.'s dental work done, including two lower bridges. They were stable for 20-plus years. A.K.'s boss did not support his sick leave for dental work, so the brothers did the best they could.

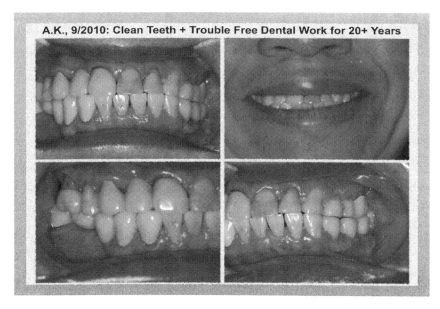

A.K., 9/2010: Clean Teeth + Trouble Free Dental Work for 20+ Years

A.K. had signs of an impaired mouth, as well: palatal asymmetry, severe tongue-tie, and a bony overgrowth on his palate, which suggests jaw clenching and teeth grinding. [2] But these clues were not part of F.K.'s dental school education, nor is SBAD a topic in any of his extensive continuing education

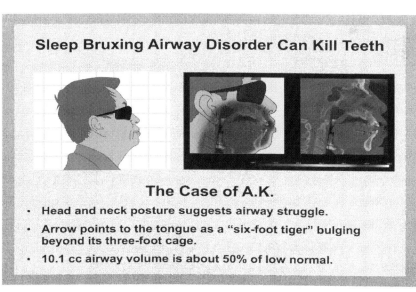

Sleep Bruxing Airway Disorder Can Kill Teeth

The Case of A.K.

- Head and neck posture suggests airway struggle.
- Arrow points to the tongue as a "six-foot tiger" bulging beyond its three-foot cage.
- 10.1 cc airway volume is about 50% of low normal.

Color scale: white = low risk of airway collapse;
red = high; black = extremely high

As soon as he recognized the connection between sleep bruxing and a narrow airway, F.K. gave A.K. an epigenetic oral appliance. A sleep test was recommended but not done because A.K. was more worried about paying for his two kids' college tuitions. He also lost his oral appliances but did not report the loss until a whole year later, when he could not drive to work because his cataract surgery had been canceled as a result of his runaway blood sugar levels.

Explaining that diabetes is beatable, starting with a new diet and exercise plan, F.K. ordered two diabetic cookbooks and instructed A.K.'s wife to cook him only the meals recommended in them. Ever since, A.K.'s fasting blood sugar has been under 90. With help from an acupuncturist and by sticking to the diet and exercise plan, he lost 50 pounds.

But while A.K.'s diabetes was under control, his sleep bruxing was not.

Once his cataract surgery was done, A.K. received his replacement oral appliance, which he misplaced yet again, but he did not make it back to his brother's office until two years later. That is when A.K. told him, "My local dentist has been fixing one tooth after another lately, and I'd like you to take a look." By that time, both of his lower bridges were gone, and he had barely enough teeth to chew with. In addition, A.K. had started wearing hearing aids in both ears, and he had begun to fret about his memory.

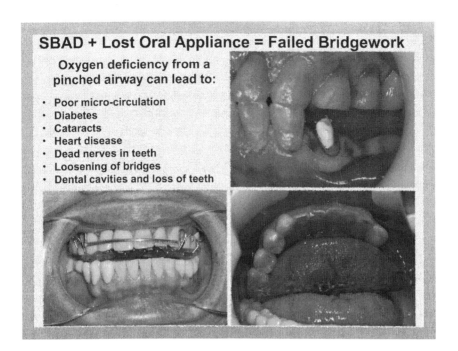

SBAD + Lost Oral Appliance = Failed Bridgework

Oxygen deficiency from a pinched airway can lead to:

- Poor micro-circulation
- Diabetes
- Cataracts
- Heart disease
- Dead nerves in teeth
- Loosening of bridges
- Dental cavities and loss of teeth

Sleep bruxing had claimed A.K.'s teeth one after another, and it's rooted in his airway — in hind sight. Recall Marie's $90,000 case earlier in this chapter. A healthy diet and exercise plan had *not* been enough. This is a costly but valuable lesson for all patients, dentists, and healthcare professionals alike.

In my opinion, the rapid progressive tooth loss was due in large part to A.K.'s airway volume of 10.6 cc – only about half of what is systemically comfortable. His brother referred him for a sleep test again and urged him to get on continuous positive airway pressure (CPAP) as soon as possible, if indicated.

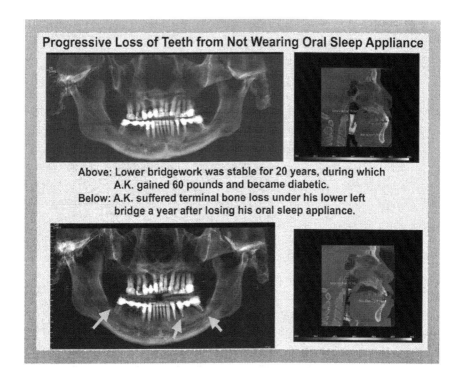

Progressive Loss of Teeth from Not Wearing Oral Sleep Appliance

Above: Lower bridgework was stable for 20 years, during which A.K. gained 60 pounds and became diabetic.
Below: A.K. suffered terminal bone loss under his lower left bridge a year after losing his oral sleep appliance.

The OSA-Diabetes Connection

Studies have provided good evidence linking obstructive sleep apnea (OSA) and diabetes. One study found that "up to 40 percent of people with OSA will have diabetes." [3]

Another found that "In people who have diabetes, the prevalence of OSA may be up to 23 percent." [4] Yet another noted, "The prevalence of some form of SDB [in diabetics] may be as high as 58 percent." [5]

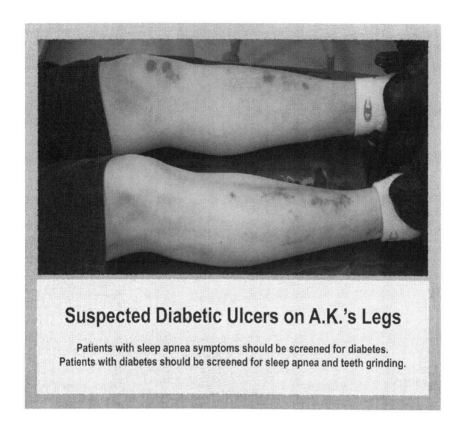

Suspected Diabetic Ulcers on A.K.'s Legs

Patients with sleep apnea symptoms should be screened for diabetes.
Patients with diabetes should be screened for sleep apnea and teeth grinding.

A.K. had both diabetes, sleep bruxing, and some memory decline. Diabetes is more likely to create bone loss under the gums, and sleep bruxing is connected to sleep disordered breathing, which in turn can result in poor microcirculation, dead nerves in teeth, failed root-canals, cracked teeth and roots, loosening of bridges, and dental cavities.

The combination of diabetes, obesity, sleeping with airway obstruction, and not wearing oral appliances can literally kill teeth.

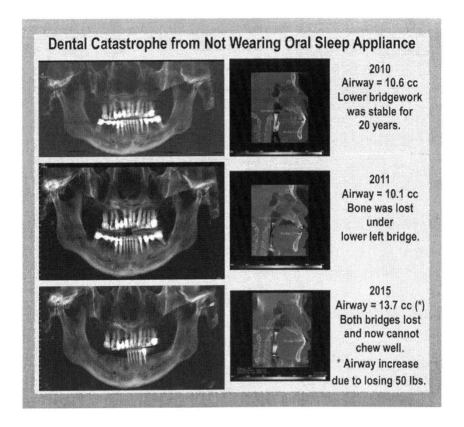

Dental Catastrophe from Not Wearing Oral Sleep Appliance

2010
Airway = 10.6 cc
Lower bridgework
was stable for
20 years.

2011
Airway = 10.1 cc
Bone was lost
under
lower left bridge.

2015
Airway = 13.7 cc (*)
Both bridges lost
and now cannot
chew well.
* Airway increase
due to losing 50 lbs.

The Case of F.K.

F.K. did biomimetic appliance therapy, as well, but with a very different outcome. The difference maker? He was true to his oral appliance, which in turn was true to his airway.

Redeveloping his impaired mouth and airway improved his airway significantly. Over three years before treatment, F.K.'s Apnea-Hypopnea Index (AHI) was 23, which is a sign of moderate OSA. Therapy reduced that to 6.1, signifying the mildest of mild OSA.

FK's Sleep Test After Biomimetic Oral Appliance Therapy

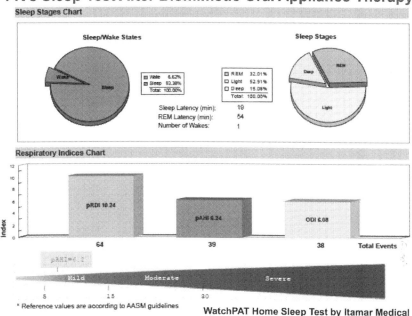

WatchPAT Home Sleep Test by Itamar Medical

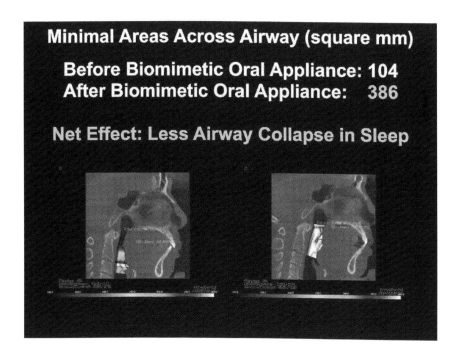

Minimal Areas Across Airway (square mm)

Before Biomimetic Oral Appliance: 104
After Biomimetic Oral Appliance: 386

Net Effect: Less Airway Collapse in Sleep

A.K.'s impaired sleep-airway-mouth brought him diabetes, dental failure and a small stroke which left him with this lasting inconvenience: "Getting dressed is a royal pain every day," he told me. "My left arm is still weak and slow!" That's about the luckiest outcome you can hope for with a stroke.

Looking back, however, an early clue on A.K.'s downhill slide was his fading memory. He could not remember had placed his appliance time and again.

Meanwhile, F.K.'s wide open airway left him productive and healthy, and his healthcare cost over the same period is less than 1% of A.K.'s. Which medical-dental-financial fate would you rather have?

A pinched airway can kill teeth, whereas a wide-open airway is the real health insurance in that the body can renew itself during sleep – as it was designed to do. The great news: pinched airway can now be redeveloped with epigenetic orthopedic oral appliances.

Holistic Mouth Nuggets

- SBAD (Sleep Bruxing Airway Disorder) is a contributing cause to many dental woes, huge dental bills, and part of Impaired Mouth Syndrome with many serious medical consequences such as diabetes and stroke.

- An impaired mouth is a predictable source of pain, fatigue, degeneration from airway obstruction and sleep troubles, Holistic Mouth is a natural solution to resolve many Impaired Mouth-related symptoms.

- The airway trumps diet and exercise. A wide-open airway is critical to aging well, and the real prize in healthcare.

Chapter 7

What Color is Your Airway? Linking Acid Reflux, Sensitive Teeth, Impaired Mouth

Sleep apnea and acid reflux go hand in hand.
— Steven Y. Park, MD, author of *Sleep Interrupted*

A narrow airway can contribute to a wide variety of health complaints beyond dental – complaints you might have been surprised to find connected with the jaw size, shape, and position, i.e., an Impaired Mouth. This extends to acid reflux (gastro-esophageal reflux disease, or GERD, which cuts across all ethnic groups and ages.

GERD happens when "an obstruction causes a vacuum effect in the throat, which suctions up your normal stomach juices into your throat, causing more inflammation and swelling, causing more obstruction." Dr. Steven Park notes that those stomach juices contain many other irritating substances, including bile, digestive enzymes, and bacteria…these are major sources of inflammation and swelling in your upper airway." [1]

Acid reflux "is the third most common gastrointestinal disorder in the U.S. and one of the leading causes of disturbed sleep among people between the ages of 45 and 64," according to the 2002 National Science Foundation *Sleep in America* poll. [2] One Hungarian study states that "sleeping can be considered as a risk factor of the reflux event by itself." [3]

Dentally, the regurgitated stomach acid can dissolve dental enamel, the hardest tissue in the body. Loss of enamel can cause exquisite sensitivity and extensive tooth damage in the presence of teeth grinding if the sleep-airway-mouth link is overlooked.

The earlier the connection of GERD, teeth damage, and sleep apnea is made, the better for the patient. Otherwise, it can be quite costly both dentally and medically, as we shall soon see in the case of T.D.

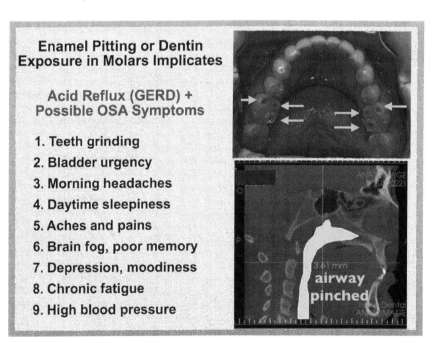

The case of T.D. Yellow arrows point to enamel pitting.

Acid Reflux and Sleep Apnea: The Dental Connection

Exquisite tooth sensitivity to brushing or cold and inflamed or receding gums are common dental concerns I hear from new patients. When I do, I also ask if they also have a sore throat or mucus that needs frequently clearing or a runny nose, post-nasal drip, or bad breath in the morning? How about heartburn, belching, chronic bronchial asthma, bronchitis, or cough? All these symptoms can be traced back to acid reflux.

Here is how the National Science Foundation describes it: "GERD describes a back flow of acid from the stomach into the esophagus.... If the acid backs up as far as the throat and larynx, the sleeper will wake up coughing and choking. If the acid only backs up as far as the esophagus the symptom is usually experienced as heartburn.... The most frequently reported symptoms of GERD are: heartburn, acid regurgitation, inflammation of the gums, erosion of the enamel of the teeth, bad breath, belching, chronic sore throat." [4]

A review from Hungary reports that "the most recognized manifestations [of GERD] are non-cardiac chest pain, bronchial asthma, chronic bronchitis, chronic cough, and posterior laryngitis, as well as the acidic damage of dental enamel." [5]

"Clinical evidence strongly suggests that GERD is associated with sleep disturbances such as shorter sleep duration, difficulty falling asleep, arousals during sleep, poor sleep quality, and awakening early in the morning," reports a 2012 study in the *Journal of Gastroenterology*. [6]

Another 2010 study found that "there is a significant association between disturbed sleep and GERD, and this may be bidirectional. Sleep disorders may induce gastrointestinal (GI) disturbances, while GI symptoms also may provoke or worsen sleep derangements." [7]

"Symptoms of OSA are possibly associated with an increased risk of Barrett's esophagus, an association that appears to be mediated entirely by gastro-esophageal reflux," reports a 2015 *PLoS ONE* study. [8] Barrett's esophagus is a precursor to cancer.

Bottom line: Acid reflux may be connected to sleep apnea, and thus not be taken lightly. Long term use of over-the-counter remedies or prescription drugs can miss or mask sleep apnea as an underlying cause and Impaired Mouth as a source.

Acid-eroded Teeth: Leading Indicator of OSA?

Normally, humans are born with enough enamel to eat and chew for a lifetime. Common enamel destroyers include: lemon sucking or tobacco chewing (rare in my office), or soda drinks containing phosphoric acid (also rarely), teeth grinding (very frequently), and acid reflux during sleep (more often than I care to see).

Pitting in the enamel, usually in the upper and lower molars are seen in old and young people alike – folks who often do not know they grind their teeth or have acid reflux. Left untreated, acid erosion continues to melt away the enamel until the sensitive layer of dentin is exposed. Dentin looks yellow-brownish compared the pearly-chalky white enamel. Dentinal exposure can be exquisitely sensitive once protective enamel coat is dissolved away.

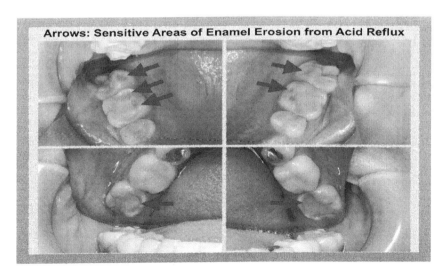

Arrows: Sensitive Areas of Enamel Erosion from Acid Reflux

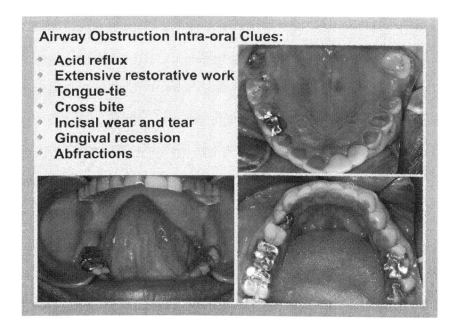

Airway Obstruction Intra-oral Clues:

* Acid reflux
* Extensive restorative work
* Tongue-tie
* Cross bite
* Incisal wear and tear
* Gingival recession
* Abfractions

Dental enamel pitting is an early indicator of sleep apnea, in my opinion, although formal research is needed. Teeth grinding and airway should be checked in the presence of enamel pitting.

The Case of T.D.

T.D. was a federal employee who had retired from a career in the U.S. military. His presenting complaints to me were erectile dysfunction, declining memory, teeth grinding, and CPAP intolerance. My examination findings included very clean teeth and gums, plus the following:

- His uvula was not visible, indicating a strong sleep apnea risk.

- His front teeth showed matching facets and fractured edges, indicating sleep bruxing.

- Misaligned upper and lower dental midlines from crossbite at his upper right lateral incisor.

- Multiple areas of gum recession, abfractions, and broken teeth, likely from teeth grinding.

- Four crowns among his upper teeth and three crowns in the lower arch

- A narrow, V-shaped upper arch suggested an underdeveloped maxilla and airway

- Severe erosion on the palatal side of all his upper teeth, indicating chronic acid reflux, a frequent sign of OSA.

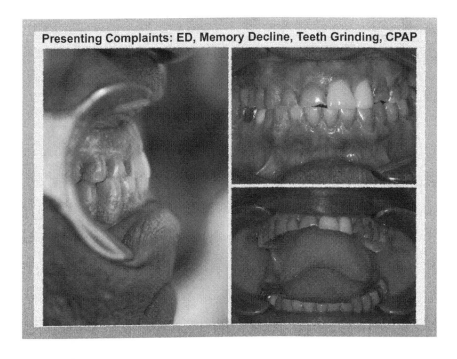

Presenting Complaints: ED, Memory Decline, Teeth Grinding, CPAP

I referred T.D. for a sleep test, which came back with a medical diagnosis of moderate OSA. CPAP had not worked so well for T.D., based on his sleep best Yet his teeth were much too damaged to start the oral appliance therapy. The tongue side of his upper teeth had been dissolved by years of nightly acid reflux from his chest heaves to free his throat of the six-foot tiger blocking his airway. He did have sound roots under those damaged teeth, but his stem cells could not be switched on until the dissolved portions of his teeth had been restored.

Medical Diagnosis: Moderate Obstructive Sleep Apnea

Interpretation

The total recording time for this polysomnogram was 398.0 minutes and the tot
58.7%. Sleep latency was 9.0 minutes and REM latency was 94.5 minutes. Sleep
sleep. **The overall Apnea Hypopnea index (AHI) was 16.0/hr.**, REM AHI was 18.6
(AI) was 6.1/hr., and the overall Hypopnea index (HI) was 9.9/hr. There were 60
apneas, 37 hypopneas, and 15 central apneas. Mean duration of events was
total of 102 arousals for an arousal index of 27.2/hr. Mean oxygen saturation w
desaturations associated with events had a nadir of 89%. Mild and intermitten
no ectopy. PLM's are within normal limits. Abnormal movements were not not

Diagnosis

Moderate Obstructive Sleep Apnea (327.23)

Could this patient have had an earlier diagnosis?

Recommendations

- Follow up with referring provider.
- Follow up consultation with sleep specialist.
- PAP titration study or dental appliance consultation to determine the
  sleep related breathing disorder.
- Maintain ideal body weight and treatment of nasal congestion or alle
- ENT evaluation.
- Precautions while driving or performing other tasks that require alertn
- The following behavioral adjustments are also recommended:

Why not just rebuild all his teeth? At the lower in-network fees, rebuilding his teeth would cost over $15,000 for 16 crowns, and his dental plan maxed out at $1,500 a year. As much as he wanted to start treatment, that stopped T.D. cold.

This is no way to treat a veteran who devoted a career to servicing our country. How did T.D get to this point?

Questions and Lessons

Did T.D. receive WholeHealth care or patchwork care? This distinction carries enormous consequences. An earlier diagnosis would have spared him the loss of three-quarters of his teeth to nightly stomach acid attacks, the damage to his heart, and sexual functions due to sleep apnea. This is the lesson from T.D.'s case.

How can we minimize cases like T.D.? What's the best way to stop the costly medical and dental care? The short answer is Impaired Mouth diagnosis, and the earlier, the better.

In my view, T.D., all his attending doctors and dentists, and all their other patients are victims of a health care system with built-in medical, dental, and mental divides that do not exist inside the body. His dentists fixed each tooth as it broke down, and his doctors treated acid reflux and sleep apnea with tunnel vision-based prescriptions. And T.D. is left with the medical and dental bills that he cannot afford to treat the root causes of his symptoms. What's wrong with this picture if you are the patient?

The solution is simple: Redeveloping an impaired mouth structurally in the direction of a Holistic Mouth as part of an overall wellness program can resolve many dental, medical, and mood symptoms effectively and without side effects. This requires WholeHealth teamwork and inter-professional outreach.

Later comments from T.D. include the following: "I was ignorant of acid reflux, sleep apnea-dental destruction and the negative results of having these issues. As a former military serviceman, I would hope that this type of healthcare is available to ALL members of the armed service in every capacity i.e. active duty, reservist, and retirees to include the family members."

A portion of the sale of this book will go to a "scholarship fund" at to help T.D. get his Holistic Mouth Solutions.

What Color Is Your Airway?

A color scale is used in CT imaging software to reflect the risk of airway collapse from the vacuum created by airway size and constriction. On the far right of the scale, white means low risk. The more the airway color is to the left of the scale, the higher the risk of airway obstruction in sleep. Keep in mind that airway is likely more closed during sleep, because office-based CT imaging is usually done with the patient standing.

This patient in her mid-20s is one of the handful of patients I have seen in the past 7 years with a healthy airway in the white zone. She will likely age well. Notice that her mouth shows a convex profile below her nose.

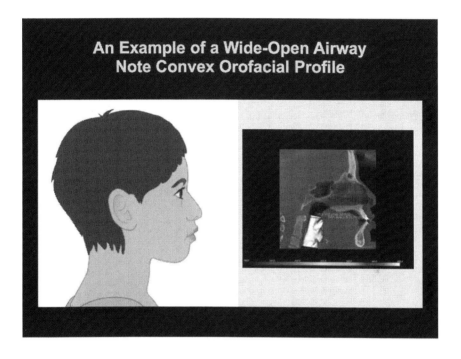

Below is C.K., a patient in his mid-40s with a history of male reproductive cancer. He found out about his airway deficiency only after chemotherapy. He is doing well after including oral appliance therapy as part of his cancer treatment. (For more on this, see Chapter 14 in *Six-Foot Tiger Three-Foot Cage*.)

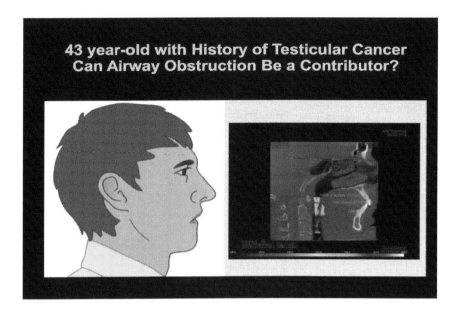

This 45-year old woman was nearly bankrupt from trying to overcome her chronic fatigue and fibromyalgia with conventional and functional medicine. She could not afford to start oral appliance therapy.

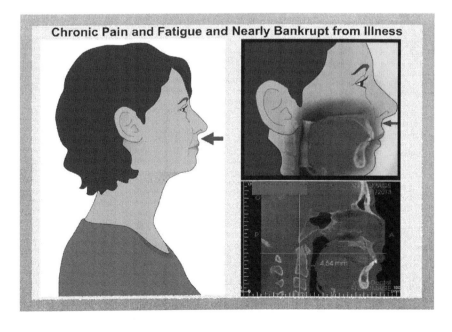

Next comes BN, a 62-year-old woman is already losing her memory and will soon lose all her teeth on her upper right side. Will dental implants work if her oral airway is off-the-color-scale narrow? More details ahead in chapter 16.

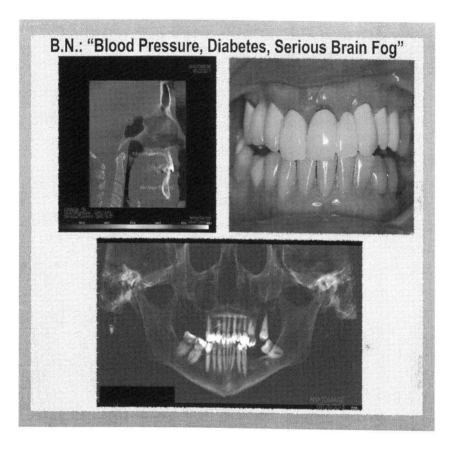

This is S.G., a new father in his early 40s who biked to work every day and had a heart attack one morning. He learned about his pinched airway and Impaired Mouth and obstructive sleep apnea only after his heart attack.

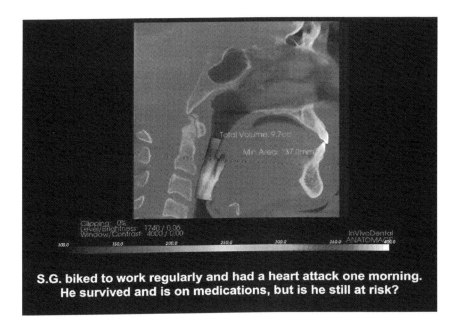

S.G. biked to work regularly and had a heart attack one morning.
He survived and is on medications, but is he still at risk?

Now compare R.H.'s airway before her oral appliance therapy, and after — see chapter 4.

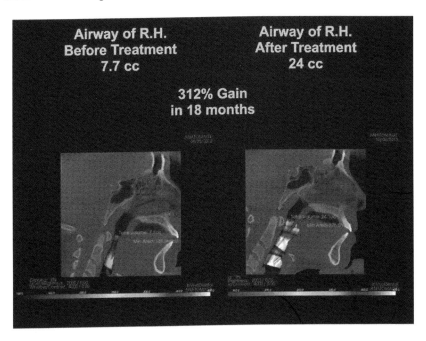

Which one of these airways would you rather have? The more the airway color is to the right, the flatter your aging trajectory. The narrower the airway, the steeper your downhill slide.

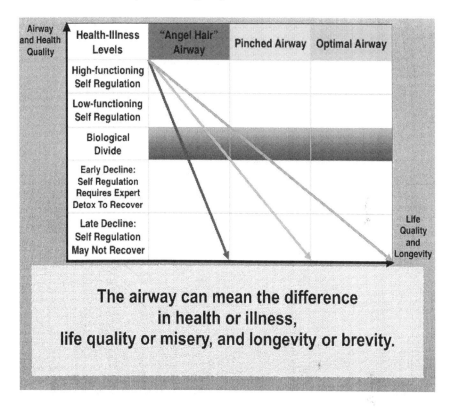

**The airway can mean the difference
in health or illness,
life quality or misery, and longevity or brevity.**

Holistic Mouth Nuggets

- Enamel pitting in molars can be an early sign of acid reflux which can result in sensitive teeth from dentinal exposure if not controlled. Acid reflux in turn is associated with sleep apnea and its global side effects.

- Know the color of your airway and choose your insurance coverage from plans that support treatment of sleep apnea, airway redevelopment, and soft-tissue support like oral-facial myofunctional therapy, cranio-sacral therapy, and training in wellness-building skill.

- The case of T.D. highlights the need to train dentists and doctors alike on oral-systemic links, including those arising from an impaired mouth and pinched airway. Lack of such education and inter-professional teamwork can cause enormous damage and costs to patients, insurers, employers, and our national treasury.

Chapter 8

You Too Can Be "Very Happy I Didn't Need Another Root-Canal!"

The mind is like a parachute — it works only when open.

– Frank Zappa

Few words strike more fear into a patient than "root-canal treatment." It is said that in old days, a mind-blowing toothache was the only acceptable excuse for breaking an appointment with a king's court.

"No root-canal for me please" is among the most frequent request I hear from new patients. Nearly all of them come with excellent dental hygiene and a history of clean medical and dental checkups for years. I also hear "I know about root-canal toxicity, and I have had too many of them. So what else can you do for my toothache?"

All too often, root-canal treatment becomes an "automatic next step" when lingering sensitivities and toothaches persist after routine dental work. Dentists have to face such worried and frustrated patients more often than they care to admit.

Can root-canals be avoided and toothaches reversed? Yes, but only sometimes, and it depends on many factors. But there is a way when the patient shows up early enough and the dentist is trained in WholeHealth.

Let's be very clear: We are NOT talking about raging toothaches from huge cavities or abscessed teeth that have ignored for too long. We are dealing with reversing dental sensitivity, nagging toothaches or bite tenderness in cavity-free teeth of recent origin.

Reversible toothache is about taking the stressors off a tooth so its comfort zone is maintained. Reversible toothache applies ONLY to cases of "this just started a day or two ago", or nagging soreness persisting after dental treatment — when the pulp is likely still alive and the blood supply to the tooth remains intact to have a shot at recovery.

A cavity needs to be cleaned out and filled, but a tooth with the same cavity but with extra stress from jaw clenching and teeth grinding may end up with symptoms after dental work.

A cavity is a bacterial invasion from dental plaque. This is the prevailing explanation for toothaches. Once pathogens have "breached the castle" and reached the nerve (pulp) in the center of the tooth, the resulting inflammation triggers the toothache, or *pulpitis*. The *-itis* ending means inflammation, and toothaches are excruciatingly painful because the inflammation is magnified within a tooth's unyielding confines. A healthy body has lot of "fire extinguishers" to put out inflammation, but a body suffering from Impaired Mouth Syndrome may not have the ability to return to normal so easily.

WholeHealth sees a bigger picture beyond the bacterial plaque. A tooth involved in teeth grinding, jaw clenching as is already traumatized and thus may not take to dental work so kindly. Add the referred pain from trigger points, which we will cover shortly, the tooth may just "go south" on you. Before we look at a case of "very happy I don't need root-canal", let's look inside a tooth to better understand this powerful source of pain.

Root Canal Anatomy: Highly Complex

"Root canals" are end branches of nerves intertwined with terminal twigs of the lymphatic and vascular tree. That's why root canal anatomy can get very complicated, as seen in the images below by Germany's Professor Walter Hess. Root-canal treatment (*endodontics*) consists of cleaning out the spaces occupied by those soft tissues and filling it with an inert material.

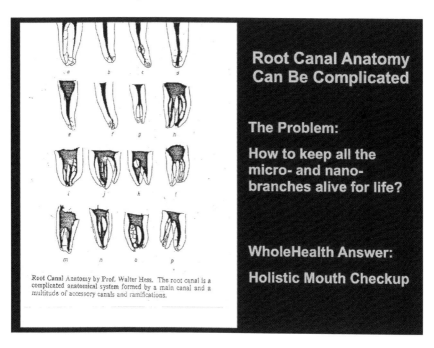

Root Canal Anatomy by Prof. Walter Hess. The root canal is a complicated anatomical system formed by a main canal and a multitude of accessory canals and ramifications.

Root Canal Anatomy Can Be Complicated

The Problem:

How to keep all the micro- and nano- branches alive for life?

WholeHealth Answer:

Holistic Mouth Checkup

Teeth that undergo root-canal treatment are often called dead teeth because their blood and nerve supply has been cut. This removes the tooth's ability to report further pain and inflammation until it goes beyond the tooth. That is why cavities in a root-canaled tooth are not felt and can destroy it fast.

The complexity of the root-canal system makes perfect-root-canal treatment highly challenging. This may explain why some teeth remain problematic after root-canal treatment.

After and Side Effects of Root-Canals

Patients with two or more root-canal treated (RCT) teeth have a 60% higher risk for heart disease, reported a 2009 study published in the *Journal of American Dental Association.* [1] Does this surprise you?

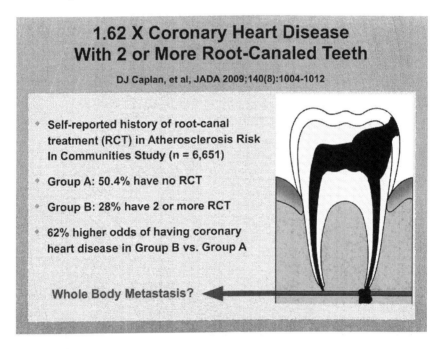

1.62 X Coronary Heart Disease With 2 or More Root-Canaled Teeth

DJ Caplan, et al, JADA 2009;140(8):1004-1012

* Self-reported history of root-canal treatment (RCT) in Atherosclerosis Risk In Communities Study (n = 6,651)

* Group A: 50.4% have no RCT

* Group B: 28% have 2 or more RCT

* 62% higher odds of having coronary heart disease in Group B vs. Group A

Whole Body Metastasis? ⬅

An evolved minority of doctors and dentists have argued that keeping a dead tooth is bad for whole body health. [2, 3, 4] Dr. George E. Meinig's *Root-canal Cover-Up* summarizes Dr. Weston A. Price's decades-long research on 5,000 animals as follows: "Root-canal-filled teeth always remain infected no matter how good they might look or how good they might feel." [5]

Dr. Thomas Levy, MD, JD, highly respected author of *Hidden Epidemic*, says, "The most current scientific literature is very clear in concluding that the pathogens typical for gum disease and root-canal-treated teeth are the direct cause for most heart attacks. The same studies also indicate a very strong likelihood that most cases of breast cancer are caused by the lymph drainage delivery of the same pathogens from such gums and teeth to the breast tissue." [6]

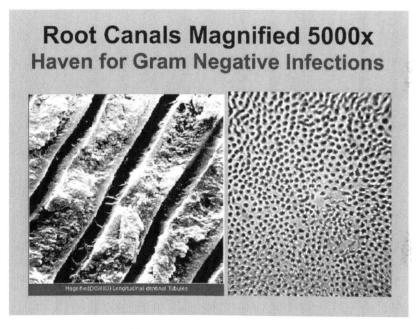

Is it possible to "sterilize and fill" every nook and cranny of the root-canal system inside a tooth?

Root-canal treated teeth do fail by the criteria of root-canal specialists (*endodontists*). The American Association of Endodontists offers an evidence-based analysis of root-canal success and failure, and the criteria for re-treatment of failed root-canals versus dental implants as the next step. [7]

The decision for root-canal treatment is an individual one, depending on the dentist, the patient, and the patient's goals. Some patients do not want to lose a single tooth, while others do not want root-canal teeth's impact on the Whole. Root-canaled teeth are the dead inside. Dead tissues in other parts of the body are surgically removed. Why should a dead tooth be any exception to the rule?

Know yourself, and know what you want and do not want, and interview your dentist and doctor for their opinion on root-canal treatment.

Common sense says that a patient who is susceptible to colds and pneumonia is more likely to have dental infections from lower immunity, which in turn is affected by sleep, nasal congestion, gut inflammation, poor diet, dysfunctional hormones, and a self-destructive lifestyle.

In my practice, the patient's overall health is as important as their dental preference. In the presence of good health, I give patient the choice: consult an endodontist, an oral surgeon, or another biological dentist. (Biological dentists have taken additional training on oral-systemic connections and integrative support on this complex issue.)

Where there is heart disease, cancer, autoimmune disease, inflammatory disease, degenerative neurological disease, and other serious body burdens, I refer the patient for medical evaluation and offer my WholeHealth view.

When there is mild or moderate inflammation or degeneration, I refer the patient for basic wellness support such as acupuncture, nutritional and lifestyle counseling as needed, and support their airway and sleep with oral appliances that suit their needs.

This was the case with Chema, who had complained of pain inside her forehead and left temple and the teeth anchoring her upper front bridge, both of which had undergone root-canal treatment. Her hospital-based neurologist had given the green light to extract those two root-canaled teeth. Chema had done her research and was mentally prepared for the extractions.

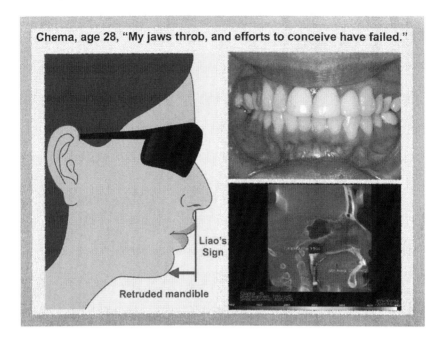

Chema, age 28, "My jaws throb, and efforts to conceive have failed."

Liao's Sign

Retruded mandible

When I evaluated her, I saw that she had a much bigger problem than her root-canaled teeth. Yes, it was her airway. She was grinding her teeth in her sleep to cope with a constricted airway, and her root-canaled teeth were paying the price.

Her pain went away within the first week of wearing an upper expander appliance for adults. Today, she is the joyous mother of a healthy one-year old baby, and she still has her bridge.

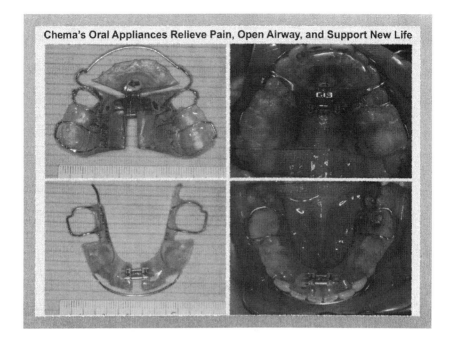

Chema's Oral Appliances Relieve Pain, Open Airway, and Support New Life

The WholeHealth Perspective

When a tooth starts to act up, see a biological dentist or Holistic Mouth Doctor right away if you wish to avoid root-canal treatment. On this point, I highly recommend Dr. Louisa Williams' article "The Importance of Acute Supportive Care in Biological Dentistry." Dr. Williams is a chiropractic and naturopathic doctor and author of an outstanding out-of-the-box book *Radical Medicine*. [8]

The WholeHealth perspective understands teeth are part of the Whole. So dental and systemic health should factor into the success/ failure of any root-canal treatment. Root-canal treatment stops the pain signal short term, but does "killing the nerve" serve the interest of whole body health?

More than three-quarters of all heart attacks involves hidden oral infection. A 2013 study in *Circulation* on the bacterial signatures in heart attack clots found that "bacterial DNA typical for endodontic infection, mainly oral viridans streptococci, was measured in 78.2% of thrombi [heart attack clots]". [9]

Is heart attack prevention one of your goals? As the ADA Council on Scientific Affairs states, "More specifically, evidence-based care means the judicious use of current best evidence, recognizing that no study is perfect in every respect or necessarily applicable to every patient." [10]

Early and Timely: Timing Is Critical for WholeHealth to Work

Root-canal treatment can be a god-send relief in the throe of a raging toothache. There is evidence that no root-canal is better if it can be avoided. The key term is *reversible pulpitis*.

Toothache happens when inflammation creates swelling or throbbing. If inflammation continues unabated, swelling can strangulate the tiny branches of the pulp to death.

Timely intervention and effective anti-inflammatory measures are critical. The window of opportunity to reverse a tooth with reversible pulpits is only a handful of days, especially in chronic bruxers with long history of Impaired Mouth Syndrome.

Since a tooth is connected to the Whole, a toothache can have more than a dental cause, and therefore more than one way to treat it. Factors such as emotional stress, diet, seasonal change, and poor posture can be aggravators. In WholeHealth, the point is to reverse toothache in its early stages, before the nerve tissue inside the tooth dies, by removing all the stressors from the tooth.

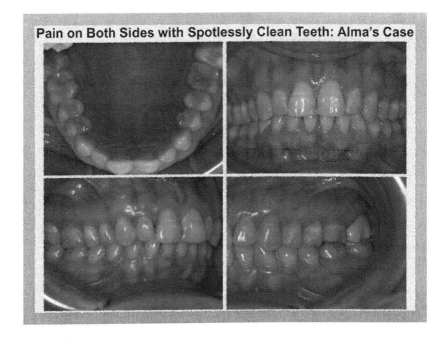

Pain on Both Sides with Spotlessly Clean Teeth: Alma's Case

Taking a WholeHealth approach here means:

- **The Holographic Truth:** That all blood to the heart, brain, and the tiniest "nerves" inside teeth all are subject to the same rules. They can be damaged by atherosclerosis, a low-mineral and high-sugar diet, high stress, oxygen deficiency, sleep apnea, snoring, and more. The smaller the blood vessel, the less leeway and the greater the risk for damage. The more jaw clenching, the more blood supply is cut off from the teeth. The narrower the airway, the stronger the jaw clenching and teeth grinding.

- **Tooth-Organ Connections:** A tooth can affect an organ through its corresponding acupuncture meridian, and vice versa. A root-canal treated tooth may correspond to a weakness or "short circuit" its meridian, according to Dr. Jerry Tennant, MD, author of Healing Is Voltage [11] For example, upper molars are on the Spleen-Stomach which mediate digestive functions and corresponds to anxiety and worrying, and lower molars correspond to Colon-Lung meridians which mediate breathing functions and emotionally relates to sadness, and judgmental criticism. [12, 13].

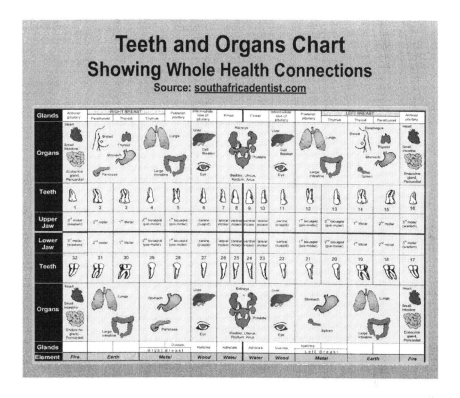

- **Holistic Mouth Solutions:** The connections between the dental "nerve" and the whole body can include circulation, nutrition, the airway, sleep, emotions, postural fascia, and the energy meridians. Holistic Mouth Solutions, as part of a WholeHealth wellness program, integrate mouth care with appropriate support from chiropractic, osteopathy, physical therapy, orofacial myofunctional therapy, acupuncture, nutrition, exercise, and stress management as needed.

WholeHealth also means making appropriate referrals to like-minded health professionals whose expertise can contribute to oral and total health.

A Tale of Two Toothaches: The Case of Alma

"I have TWO toothaches now," said Alma, a new patient who came eleven days after having two upper left fillings replaced due to constant food-packing between them. "One is on the upper left, where the new fillings are, but now I also have a toothache on my upper right, the UNTREATED side. My teeth were fine until the third day after treatment."

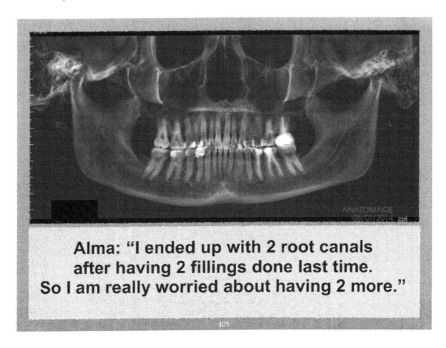

Alma: "I ended up with 2 root canals after having 2 fillings done last time. So I am really worried about having 2 more."

"That's very interesting because most toothaches do not cross midlines. Your new fillings seem fine, and I don't find any high spots. Have you had a cold recently? That can affect your sinuses. How's your stress level these days?"

"No cold and flu recently, but funny you should ask. My stress has been going through the roof. My mom has cancer, and she has just moved in with us."

"Have you been clenching your jaws and grinding your teeth?"

"Yes," said Alma.

"It's possible that your toothache maybe coming from trigger points in your shoulders and upper back activated by your streosss."

"What's that, and how so?"

Trigger Points: Toothache from a Distant Source

"Dr. Janet Travell was the doctor who successfully treated President John Kennedy's back pain. She wrote a classic textbook called the *Trigger Point Manual.* [14] 'Trigger point' means that the pain is at a site distant from its source. The pain is where the bullet lands, but the trigger is somewhere else."

"You mean my toothache isn't actually from my teeth?"

"It's possible. Look at these illustrations and see if you have the same areas. The highlighted X's are the sources of referred pain called trigger points. The shaded areas are where "the bullet lands" and where pain shows up. The *trapezius* muscle is a trapezoidal-shaped muscle attached from the mid-back of the head to the shoulder points to the mid-back. It serves to balance the head over the neck. It's the most frequent area of soreness not only because of daily stress, but also because forward head posture is a stress-inducer."

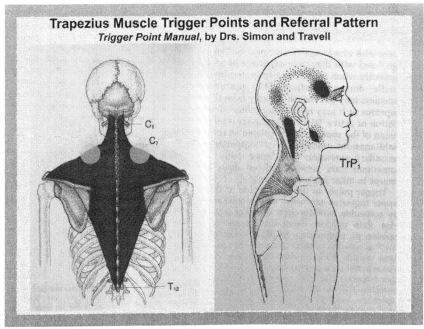

Trapezius Muscle Trigger Points and Referral Pattern
Trigger Point Manual, by Drs. Simon and Travell

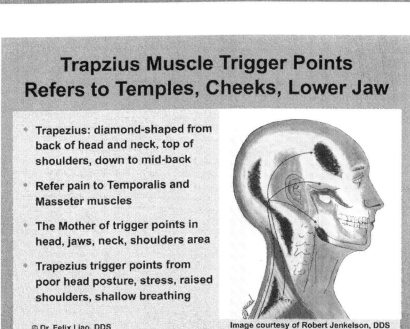

Trapzius Muscle Trigger Points
Refers to Temples, Cheeks, Lower Jaw

- Trapezius: diamond-shaped from back of head and neck, top of shoulders, down to mid-back

- Refer pain to Temporalis and Masseter muscles

- The Mother of trigger points in head, jaws, neck, shoulders area

- Trapezius trigger points from poor head posture, stress, raised shoulders, shallow breathing

© Dr. Felix Liao, DDS   Image courtesy of Robert Jenkelson, DDS

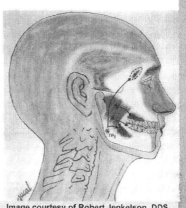

Masseter Muscle Trigger Points
Refers to Upper and Lower Molars

- Masseter: jaw-clenching muscles in front of both ears

- Trigger points refer pain and tenderness to molars

- Very common pattern

- Masseter trigger points origin: teeth grinding, and/or narrow airway, and Trapezius muscle

- Trapezius trigger points from poor head posture

© Dr. Felix Liao, DDS   Image courtesy of Robert Jenkelson, DDS

Images courtesy of Robert Jenkelson, DDS, Neuromuscular Dentistry [15]

"That's me alright, and that one, too," Alma said.

"Yes, that is a very frequent pattern in my experience." My examination confirmed the trigger points on the top of her shoulders and the "nutcracker" muscles in front of her ears.

"I want try anything that'd save me from more root-canals." Alma said, then added, "Oh, and I *have* had a history of bad TMJ. The specialist I saw wanted me to wear the appliance 24/7 for six months. I tried that, and I think that's what caused my previous root-canals."

"It's possible, but I think it's just as likely your meridians are blocked. In Traditional Chinese Medicine, meridians are channels for energy (*Chi*) flow. Like a stagnant river, meridian blockage breeds pain and illness. Do you want anti-inflammatory medications, or do you prefer a natural approach for your toothache?"

"I'd do anything to avoid root-canals, and I prefer to avoid medication. And yes, I believe in WholeHealth." With that directive from Alma, I referred her to a Whole Health acupuncturist, and her teeth have lived on without ache ever after.

Alma returned to me one week after our first appointment. She had a big smile. "I am very happy that I didn't need another root-canal. My toothaches were gone right after seeing the WholeHealth acupuncturist you suggested." Alma admitted, "The last time I had a toothache, I ended up with two root-canals."

If Columbus had not kept his mind open, he would not have discovered America. Alma kept her mind open and found an unexpected solution to her toothaches.

Impaired Mouth Raises Root-canal Risk

After Alma's initial toothaches were solved, a Holistic Mouth Checkup revealed pain on both jaw joints and tongue-tie. She was 30 pounds overweight from thyroid gland removal 14 years earlier and could not sleep through the night without waking up several times. Her airway was in the red danger zone. Due to financial constraints, she continued to live with an impaired mouth and pinched airway. But she has not needed root-canal treatment since she started seeing the WholeHealth acupuncturist.

Alma has learned how to take better care of herself and her family from her Whole Health acupuncturist — all from seeking a holistic way to fix her toothache. As the Taoist teaching says, "Give a man a fish, and you feed him for one meal. Teach a man how to fish, and you feed him for a lifetime." She now knows how to rebalance herself with healing exercises at home whenever she has any aches and pain.

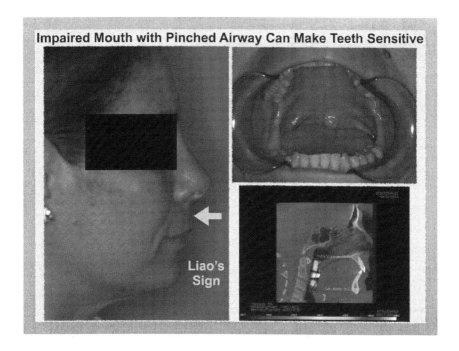

Impaired Mouth with Pinched Airway Can Make Teeth Sensitive

Liao's Sign

In my experience, an Impaired Mouth with pinched airway raises the risk of dental sensitivities, toothaches, and thus root-canal treatment recommendations. When inflammation and stress on teeth are recognized early and treated with Holistic Mouth Solutions in collaboration with WholeHealth-minded integrative health professionals, toothaches have a chance to reverse naturally.

Alma's case shows how all the oral-systemic connections are two-way streets: Teeth can hurt the neck and shoulders, and vice versa. While oral appliance therapy would have targeted a main source of Alma's pain, non-dental contributions to toothaches can be managed by "emptying the bucket" periodically through other channels, such as the low-inflammation diet her WholeHealth acupuncturist recommended. She also learned self-healing exercises to compensate for the toothache that returns when her stress gets out of control.

If you already have one root-canaled treatment and do not want another, getting a Holistic Mouth Checkup can be helpful to see if your mouth structure is an anatomical source.

A Holistic Mouth Checkup is also a good idea if you wish to proactively avoid non-cavity toothaches, persistent sensitivity, chipped teeth requiring crowns, cracked roots resulting in extractions, costly restorations, and other dental consequences of Impaired Mouth Syndrome. To see if you might benefit, take the self-survey at the end of this book to get your Impaired Mouth Syndrome score.

Holistic Mouth Nuggets

- Toothaches can have dental causes or bodily causes. Patients with Impaired Mouth and a pinched airway are more likely to have toothaches of non-dental origin.

- Not all toothaches are caused by infections, especially in patients with excellent oral hygiene, sensible diet, and healthy lifestyle. In their early stages, such toothaches can be reversed. And "early" is best time to do this — before the blood supply and the oxygen supply are shut off.

- WholeHealth not only means every part of the body is connected, but also that there is more than one way to treat a symptom or resolve a toothache. A tooth inside an Impaired Mouth with pinched airway has a higher risk of dental sensitivities, toothaches, and thus higher likelihood to receive root-canal treatment.

Chapter 9

WholeHealth Care — Putting Common Sense Back into Medical and Dental Practices

The significant problems we face cannot be solved at the same level of thinking we were at when we created them.

– Albert Einstein (attributed)

We have seen how an impaired sleep-airway-mouth link can cause pain and kill teeth. Soon we will see how it can harm the heart and the brain. Bridging the two is a WholeHealth philosophy to connect all parts of the body, including the brain, heart, as a functional and self-renewing Whole.

Health is a state of physical, emotional, nutritional, and mental well-being *in balance*, with contributions from all parts of the body. Symptoms are reactions to balance-disrupting causes, and those causes can perpetuate symptoms if not removed. Finding and treating causes can help the body heal itself naturally. Finding Impaired Mouth as a cause can actualize fuller genetic potential, renew vigor, save teeth, and bring on facial radiance, as we have seen.

The human body is amazing *and* amazingly complex. It is understandable that medical science started with reduction   that is, breaking the Whole into parts through dissection, microscopes, and molecular studies. Treatments evolved along the way with varying effectiveness. Yet many patients get sent to a specialist for each problematic body part and never feel wholly well.

WholeHealth integration is the solution.

From Parts to the Whole – and to WholeHealth

WholeHealth is the common sense that all parts of the body are connected to each other, and to our environment, the cosmos, and the Great Spirit. Your body is one complete package, in which all parts are linked and mutually supportive, and all systems are seamlessly coordinated.

But that's not how healthcare is delivered in America in 2017. Based on my patients' experience, what they have been getting is fragmented, patchwork care based on a silo mentality of specialties, fixing parts only when they hurt or cause problems.

WholeHealth, in contrast, is about connecting the body's inner environment to the outer, and mind-body-mouth-airway to Nature's laws governing health and life. The proverbial elephant is not just the sum of trunk, ears, tail, legs, and tusks. It is a unified living being that can walk, run, eat, drink, communicate, move, rest, and renew itself with sleep — as long as Impaired Mouth is a built-in source of health troubles.

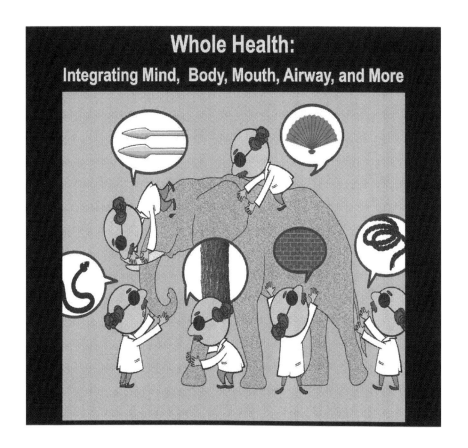

Inside the body, there are no medical, dental, nutritional, or emotional departmental lines, nor special interest turf wars, nor labels of conventional or alternative health care. But that is not how healthcare is done in America today, and patients are suffering the consequences. While the division of labor is necessary to develop expertise over all parts of the body, you have already seen what can happen to patients when dentists do only teeth, doctors do only mind and body, and the mouth is left out between the two worlds.

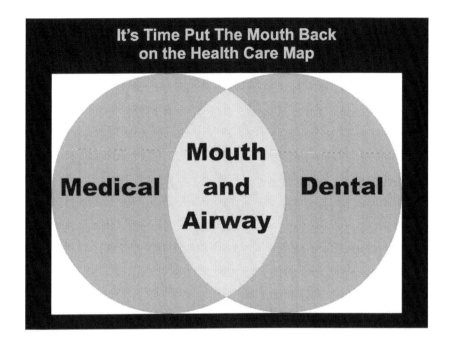

It's Time Put The Mouth Back
on the Health Care Map

Medical Mouth and Airway Dental

The "health" in WholeHealth is the outcome of teamwork to build up the Whole — teamwork inside the body, and teamwork among all your healthcare professionals. Are all the parts creating a symphony or screaming sirens? Are your organs and systems making or draining energy?

If all your body parts are connected, then EVERY part matters, from your appendix to wisdom teeth to a hair-sized root-canals in all your teeth. No room for wisdom teeth should not be an automatic justification for extractions. In the WholeHealth view, the question is WHY: why isn't there room on the bus for this late comer? Can the jaws be redeveloped so there's room for every tooth? If not, then why? If yes, then what can be done? *This* is WholeHealth inquiry transcending the dental silo.

WholeHealth is a way of seeing each patient not simply as a sum of the parts but also a blend of mind, body, mouth, emotions, family, society, and environment all blended together like a smoothie, or a mess, as each case may be.

WholeHealth takes a systems engineer's approach to see how (A) each part fits into the whole body, (B) the Whole affects individual parts, and (C) changing one part can affect others.

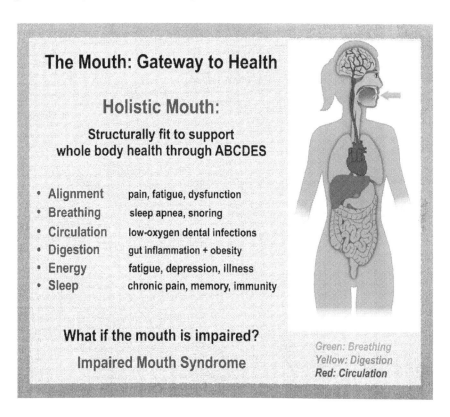

The Mouth: Gateway to Health

Holistic Mouth:

**Structurally fit to support
whole body health through ABCDES**

* Alignment   pain, fatigue, dysfunction
* Breathing   sleep apnea, snoring
* Circulation   low-oxygen dental infections
* Digestion   gut inflammation + obesity
* Energy   fatigue, depression, illness
* Sleep   chronic pain, memory, immunity

What if the mouth is impaired?

Impaired Mouth Syndrome

Green: Breathing
Yellow: Digestion
Red: Circulation

WholeHealth Starts with Holistic Mouth Solutions™

WholeHealth can mean better clinical outcome if all health professionals know more about the red book in the next slide: a structurally-impaired mouth can be the first domino leading to an inevitable syndrome of oral-systemic symptoms. It's time the dots get connected by doctors and therapists of all specialties and licenses.

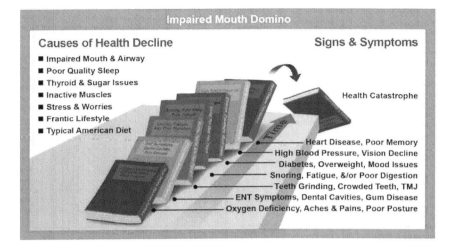

The same WholeHealth logic holds true for the cure: Holistic Mouth is a natural solution for Impaired Mouth Syndrome — without side effects or pain.

Chances are good that your dentists were not looking at your overall health when you were growing up, and your doctors these days are not looking into your mouth and checking your dental history. The medical-dental divide they were taught through their schooling persists in the way they see your symptoms and treatment.

A WholeHealth orientation can free doctors from the confines of their specialized training and all healthcare professionals from licensure limitations by allowing them to see the patient as an integrated Whole. A WholeHealth professional is aware that snoring, sleep bruxing, and related symptoms are early warning signs of sleep apnea ahead and consequent systemic damage. This awareness empowers a WholeHealth professional to guide patients toward proactive care of sleep apnea — no matter if she/he is a nurse, massage therapist, nutritionist, acupuncturist, physical therapist, physician assistant, dental hygienist, doctor of any degree.

A WholeHealth professional can suggest a Holistic Mouth Checkup whenever you have medical, dental, or mental-mood symptoms. Removing Impaired Mouth as a perpetuating factor can only help your healthcare professionals to take better care of you. You can check out your Impaired Mouth Syndrome Score in the Appendix.

The Case of Darby: "Just hurry it up a bit before I die!"

"My goal is to avoid the CPAP mask," Darby told me. "Too many of my friends have them and they hate it."

In his mid-50s, Darby came in with a distrust of doctors and dentists due to prior traumatic experience. He had taken to educating himself and realized the burdens inside his body from a lifetime of the Standard American Diet (SAD) and a long history of exposure to pesticides, phthalates, lead solders, mercury, and chlordane. He had been detoxing himself for the past ten years. "I am so much healthier now compared to before."

But he still was not where he wanted to be. His presenting concerns included high blood pressure "resistant to everything I've thrown at it," Other symptoms troubling him included lack of calm and peace of mind, generalized mouth discomfort, an embarrassing smile, and a desire for better physical fitness.

Dentally, Darby had two very loose teeth that were tender to eat with. He had lots of tartar from many years of avoiding dentists. Nine teeth were already missing. I told him that periodontal health would be foundational for Holistic Mouth Solutions to address all of his concerns.

Strong as he was intellectually and tough as he talked on the outside, Darby was paralyzed emotionally by the thought of drill-and-fill dentistry. It took a few painless treatment experiences to reprogram his mind before he could accept having his Impaired Mouth Syndrome evaluated for treatment.

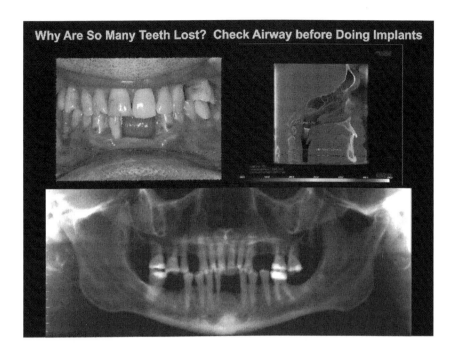

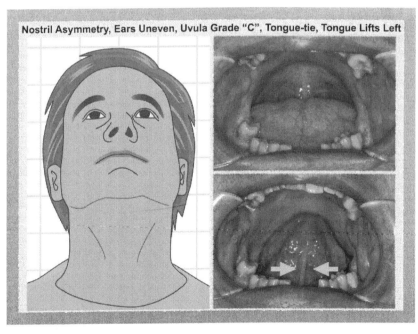

How did a smart and strong-willed man to lose nine teeth? One look at his face led me to suspect a pinched airway behind his soft palate and tongue, which was confirmed by a CT scan and a Holistic Mouth checkup.

Our CSI – Chair Side Investigation – told even more of the story behind Darby's symptoms:

- A moderate tongue-tie (see the yellow arrows in the previous slide) led to an under-developed maxilla.

- Nasal obstruction and a deviated septum contributed to part-time mouth breathing, especially during sleep.

- A retruded and deficient maxilla combined with habitual mouth breathing to start a cascade of developmental "left turns" that ended with a severely choked airway.

Sleep had thus become a life-threatening event for Darby. The tongue's habitat was too small, so it obstructed the airway, leading to oxygen deficiency. So his body was constantly experiencing a fight or flight stress response during sleep, contributing to the resistant high blood pressure.

I sent Darby for a sleep test, and told him that he would need to put in the necessary physical, mental, and financial effort to upgrade his overall health by straightening his mouth, i.e., turning his Impaired Mouth into a Holistic Mouth. He would need to wear oral appliances from sunset to sunrise and an oral-face mask during sleep. He would also need cranio-sacral therapy, myofunctional therapy, physical therapy, and lessons in breathing and posture.

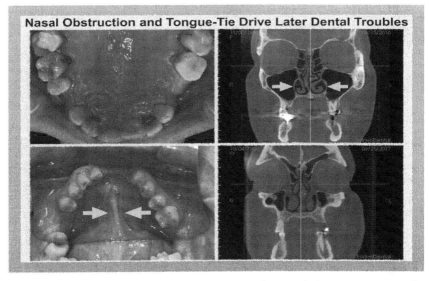

Lower left: arrows point to tongue-tie. Lower right: nasal obstruction. Top right: green arrows point to patent nasal passage. Black is airway, and gray is tissue.

"I am already gluten-, dairy-, sugar-, caffeine- and alcohol-free. I am looking forward to experiencing this Holistic Mouth process and discussing the treatment plan that you have developed. Just hurry it up a bit before I die!"

Darby later admitted that he had seen another dentist before coming to me. "Your WholeHealth philosophy appealed to me," he smiled. "Now just hurry up with my oral appliance before I die."

Patchwork Care: Frustrating and Costly

Patchwork care is fine for dealing with an emergency or crisis, such as a broken leg, heart attack, or severe toothache. Yet as people are living longer and wanting natural health and wellness, patchwork care is not so good at stopping premature degeneration and troublesome aging.

Night guards are the shining example of patchwork care in dentistry. Its use was understandable before research suggested that teeth grinding may actually be a response to airway blockage and oxygen deprivation. But today, it is a stop-gap measure at best, aiming to minimize damage. The trouble with nigh guards is that it leaves Sleep Bruxing Airway Disorder (see chapter 3) unaddressed.

And even though the connection between gum inflammation and heart disease is well-established and old news today [1, 2, 3, 4, 5], nearly all new patients tell me that no physician or holistic health professional has ever looked in their mouths — with potentially important consequences, as my patient S.H. could tell you next.

WholeHealth Is Common Sense Not Practiced: Hacking Cough Resolved with Dental Care

S.H. had come from seven states away for a second opinion. He said, "My teeth are so bad that my dentist is saying that they should all be pulled — excuse my cough — but I want to get your holistic view."

"Thank you for your confidence. Do you see your dentist regularly?"

"Yes, every six months for thirty years now."

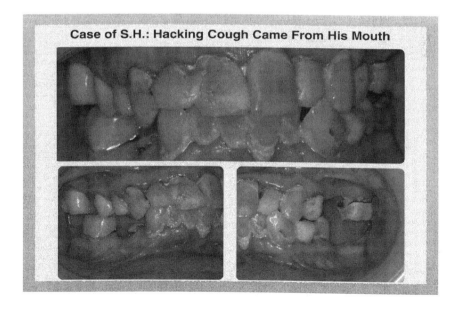

Case of S.H.: Hacking Cough Came From His Mouth

"So why are you suddenly looking at full-mouth extractions? Was there a precipitating event?"

"It's a long story. My wife came down with a disabling disease three years ago, and I've had to take over kitchen duties. It's all been very stressful." S.H. had to cough between sentences. "Then I found a brand of brownie mix that I can make myself, and I'm quite fond of it."

"How long have you had that cough, and what you have done for it?"

"I can't remember, but it came on gradually, and it's getting worse. I have been put on antibiotics, antihistamines, antacids, and steroids — you name it. Nothing has worked."

A look inside his mouth showed that it was full of grungy plaque and decay. It took from 11 am to 3 pm to clean and fill his decayed teeth. His cough stopped by the time he was leaving. "I recommend you ease off those brownies. You can eat them as dessert, but not as snacks. And do brush the leftovers off your teeth right away if you want to keep your own teeth."

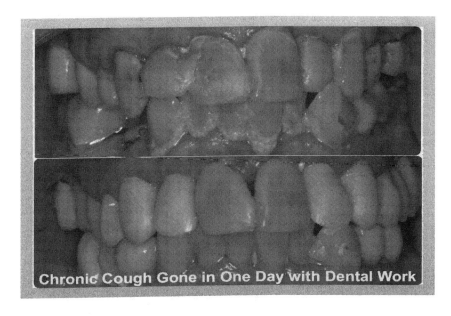

Chronic Cough Gone in One Day with Dental Work

It is fair to say that S.H.'s hacking cough was a self-defense against the teeming bacteria feeding on the brownies left over on his teeth and gums. Medications did not fix the source of his cough. Addressing his dental situation did.

"Just think of all those medications I took!" S.H. shook his head as he was leaving. Common sense would have said "Go see the dentist first" – if only his doctors had thought to look into his mouth.

WholeHealth: Mind, Body, and Mouth Integration

In summary, WholeHealth is a philosophy that follows Nature's logic governing health and life to help the body run and fix itself. WholeHealth is a platform on which physicians, dentists, all health professionals, and insurance carriers can help patients restore and maintain whole body health by acting upon these truths:

- All parts of the body are connected to one another and to Nature's laws.

- The Whole is made of all physical, emotional, fluid, and energetic systems to support healthy functions and life.

- Each part contributes to the Whole, while the Whole supports each part.

- The mouth is pivotal part of the Whole that can either build or block natural health.

- An impaired mouth handicaps the Whole's ability to run itself, which has whole body consequences.

- A holistic mouth is the start of whole body health, and a wide-open airway from a well-developed cranial-facial skeleton is a necessary part of an overall wellness program.

- Holistic Mouth Solutions can turn an impaired mouth into a Holistic Mouth to relieve or resolve many medical, dental, and mood symptoms naturally.

These statements make intuitive and scientific sense on paper. In practice, however, many patients are left hanging between the medical and dental planets.

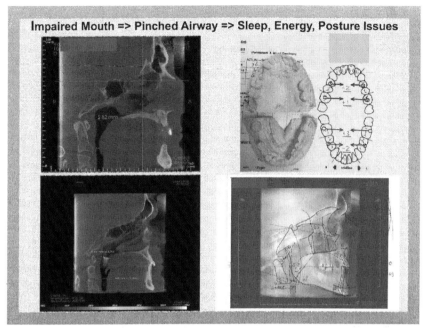

An airway that is off-the-scale deficient means higher risk for heart disease despite this patient's valiant effort at eating organic and heart-healthy.

Holistic Mouth Nuggets

- WholeHealth sees the mind, body, and mouth as one unified package, not three separate entities. It connects symptom(s) to source(s) across departmental and specialty lines. Consider WholeHealth integration and Holistic Mouth checkup when patchwork care has not worked.

- It is time to put the mouth back where it belongs in health care — in the control tower, at the start of the digestive system, in direct contact with the circulation system, and a potential choke point in the breathing system.

- Does your dentist ask about your sleep, medical history, look at your head posture, or check your Impaired Mouth

Syndrome score? Do your non-dental healthcare providers ask you about your sleep, dental history, look into your mouth, or check your Impaired Mouth Syndrome score? This is one way to tell if they are WholeHealth oriented.

Chapter 10

Hidden Heart Attack Risk Revealed by Holistic Mouth Checkup

I thought feeling sleepy during the day and waking up feeling tired were very common sleep problems, but now after reading this article I think I should not neglect them. Thanks a lot for one more nice post.

– Comment on Dr. Liao's Whole Health Blog [1]

Heart disease is America's leading killer, and the mouth is the major contributor to heart disease through not only diet, but also sleep apnea from pinched airway inside an Impaired Mouth. This heart-airway-mouth connection deserves more recognition as a source of heart disease symptoms. [2, 3]

Leading Causes of Death, 2015
Dr. Liao: choked airway, diet, and stress are major causes

1. Heart disease	23%
2. Cancer	22%
3. Chronic lower respiratory diseases	5%
4. Accidents (unintentional injuries)	5%
5. Stroke (cerebrovascular diseases)	5%
6. Alzheimer's disease	3%
7. Diabetes	3%
8. Influenza and pneumonia	2%
9. Kidney diseases	2%
10. Intentional self-harm (suicide)	2%

US Centers for Disease Control & Prevention
http://www.cdc.gov/nchs/fastats/leading-causes-of-death.htm

Asymptomatic atherosclerosis is the hardening of the arteries that you cannot feel until it's dangerously late. As the Society for Heart Attack Prevention and Eradication notes, "In over 50 percent of victims, the first symptom of asymptomatic atherosclerosis is sudden cardiac death or acute MI [myocardial infarction, or heart attack]." [4]

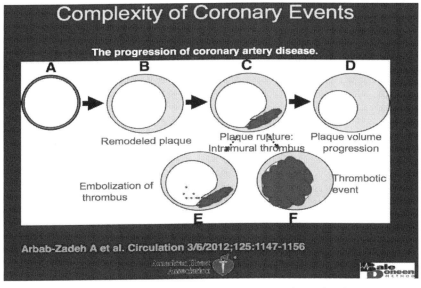

Slide courtesy of Amy Doneen, DNP, ARNP, and Brad Bale MD

So, what can you do to prevent heart disease from killing you? Besides talking to your doctor, several oral-systemic links are in your control:

a. Eat a heart-healthy diet and exercise for 3.5 hours or more a week. [5]

b. Keep your teeth in good repair and gums clean so they are not a health liability [6, 7]

c. Get a Holistic Mouth Checkup to assess the all-important sleep-airway-mouth connection to sleep apnea. [8]

Of these, Holistic Mouth checkup is the most important, in my opinion, and the most overlooked.

The patients who seek me out have generally done well on the first two items, but they still have multiple symptoms such as dental sensitivities, toothaches, teeth grinding, high blood pressure, depression, and anxiety, which can be connected to their airway and sleep.

The heart is more stressed when the airway is clogged by the tongue and the whole body is turning blue. Oxygen is absolutely the number one nutritional requirement, in my view.

Connecting Heart Attack, Undiagnosed Sleep Apnea, Impaired Mouth, Pinched Airway

S.G. was among the lucky to survive his heart attack. As his wife tells it, his "heart condition became apparent when he had a heart attack at age 43."

He was and remains relatively fit, active, and otherwise healthy, but has a very strong family history of hypertension. Once Dr. Liao educated us about the direct link between heart disease and obstructive sleep apnea, I began to realize that I could actually hear my husband struggling to take breaths throughout the night. In addition, I have noticed that if he lies down at any time of day, he is asleep within minutes.

He regularly sleeps for hours on the weekends, even after getting what appears to be a full night's sleep on weekdays. I became very concerned that he was not getting enough oxygen throughout the night, and finally he had a sleep study done at Dr. Liao's urging. He was diagnosed with moderate obstructive sleep apnea as Dr. Liao had suspected.

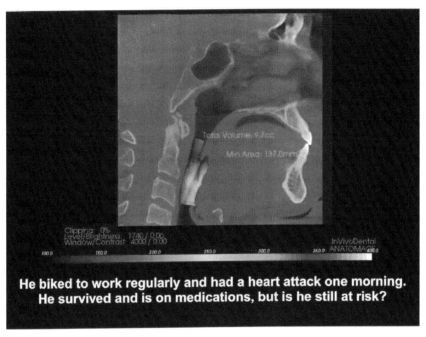

He biked to work regularly and had a heart attack one morning. He survived and is on medications, but is he still at risk?

Low normal of pharyngeal airway volume is 20 cc. S.G. had an airway of under 10 cc.

Heart attack prevention has many parts, including diet, exercise, and stress reduction. Now we can add dental visits as valuable opportunities to screen for sleep apnea and reduce heart attack risk. Holistic Mouth Checkup to evaluate mouth structure, airway, and sleep.

Long before OSA results in a heart attack or sleep bruxing destroys teeth, a Holistic Mouth Checkup by a trained health professional can help save teeth, the heart, and the brain. Let's take a closer look at

S.G.'s case, which offers valuable clues and lessons for connecting sleep bruxing with sleep apnea and heart disease.

Chair Side Investigation™: Findings from S.G.'s Holistic Mouth Checkup

S.G. was a hardworking lawyer who liked to exercise and biked to work. He had a heart attack as he arrived at his office one morning. He and his wife were expecting their first child. Despite his physical fitness, S.G. was at risk for his heart attack from the WholeHealth view linking sleep-airway-mouth-sleep apnea.

Not long before his heart attack, S.G. Said during a checkup and cleaning, "I have a broken tooth" . Before fixing it, my examination showed that S.G. had periodontal inflammation and bone loss, huge tori (bony outgrowths on the inside of the lower jaw or on the palate in response to jaw clenching and teeth grinding), and matching wear facets on his front teeth indicative of teeth grinding. His uvula was not visible when he opened his mouth, putting him at higher risk for OSA. [9, 10]

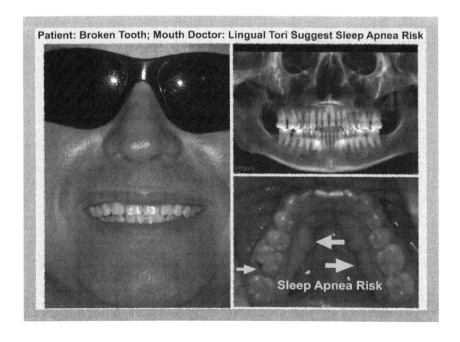

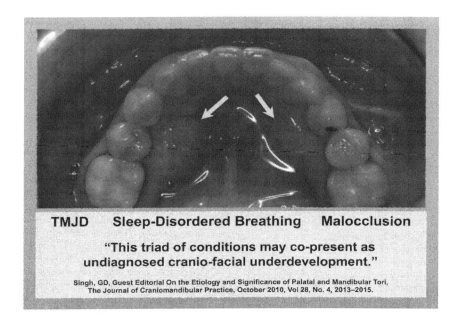

TMJD   Sleep-Disordered Breathing   Malocclusion

"This triad of conditions may co-present as
undiagnosed cranio-facial underdevelopment."

Singh, GD, Guest Editorial On the Etiology and Significance of Palatal and Mandibular Tori,
The Journal of Craniomandibular Practice, October 2010, Vol 28, No. 4, 2013–2015.

I suspected airway constriction from physical evaluation, and recommended a 3D cone-beam computed tomography (CBCT) scan because "3-dimensional CBCT airway analysis could be used as a tool to assess the presence and severity of OSA." [11]

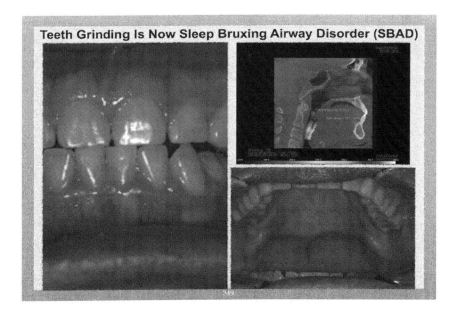

Teeth Grinding Is Now Sleep Bruxing Airway Disorder (SBAD)

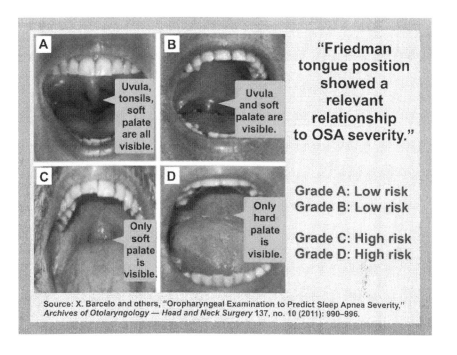

"Friedman tongue position showed a relevant relationship to OSA severity."

A: Uvula, tonsils, soft palate are all visible.
B: Uvula and soft palate are visible.
C: Only soft palate is visible.
D: Only hard palate is visible.

Grade A: Low risk
Grade B: Low risk
Grade C: High risk
Grade D: High risk

Source: X. Barcelo and others, "Oropharyngeal Examination to Predict Sleep Apnea Severity," *Archives of Otolaryngology — Head and Neck Surgery* 137, no. 10 (2011): 990–996.

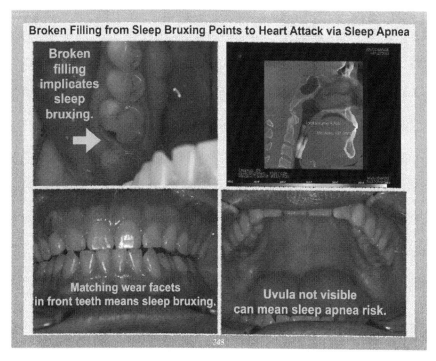

Broken Filling from Sleep Bruxing Points to Heart Attack via Sleep Apnea

Broken filling implicates sleep bruxing.

Matching wear facets in front teeth means sleep bruxing.

Uvula not visible can mean sleep apnea risk.

I referred S.G. for a sleep test to rule out Obstructive Sleep Apnea (OSA) as heart attack risk factor. After pleading busy-ness with work and admitting to fatigue, S.G. finally agreed to have it done after three years of urging between his wife and myself. During that time, S.G.'s airway had narrowed from 4.5 mm to 2.5 mm, putting him at greater risk for major adverse coronary and cerebrovascular events (MACCEs).

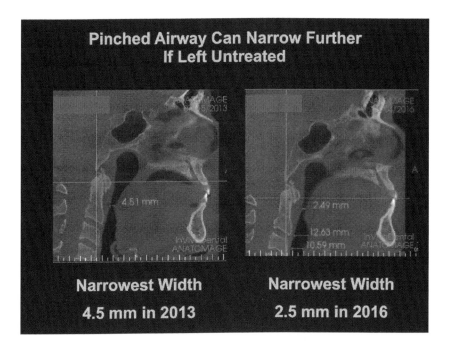

It was no surprise, then, that his diagnosis came back as moderate obstructive sleep apnea.

S.G.'s Sleep Test: AHI = 19.1

Diagnosis: Moderate Obstructive Sleep Apnea

RESPIRATORY EVENTS: The polysomnogram revealed a presence of 0 apneas resulting in an Apnea index of 0.0 events per hour. There were 96 hypopneas resulting in a Hypopnea index of 19.1 events per hour. Hypopneas are defined as a 30% reduction in airflow with an associated 3% SaO2 desaturation and/or an EEG arousal. **The overall AHI was 19.1.**

OXYGEN: Baseline oxygen saturation was 94.0%. The lowest oxygen saturation was 88.2%.

LIMB ACTIVITY: There were 174 limb movements recorded. Of this total, 140 were classified as PLMs. Of the PLMs, 1 were associated with arousals. The Limb Movement index was 34.6 per hour while the PLM index was 27.8 per hour.

CARDIAC SUMMARY: The average pulse rate was 71.2 bpm. The minimum pulse rate was 58.0 bpm while the maximum pulse rate was 102.0 bpm. No EKG abnormalities were noted.

Interpretation: This is a diagnostic study and the patient presented with moderate obstructive sleep apnea, which was exacerbated during supine sleep. Snoring was noted.

Diagnosis: Moderate obstructive sleep apnea

Recommendations:
1. Follow up with referring physician to discuss study results and treatment options.
2. Return to the sleep lab for a CPAP titration study.
3. Risk factor modification including weight loss, avoiding alcohol and sedatives and positional therapy if indicated.
4. Do not drive or operate machinery while sleepy or fatigued.

After several consultations, S.G. felt he could not be compliant with oral appliance therapy, despite his wife's wish, and continued to explore his options. They know that I will continue to be a resource and sounding board for both of them, no matter his final decision on treatment.

Airway Obstruction Links Heart Disease and Sleep Bruxing

Teeth grinding can come from mental-emotional stress. It can also come from airway distress during sleep. Can heart disease and sleep bruxing be connected? I believe yes, and here is a small sample of the evidence connecting sleep bruxing to heart disease via OSA:

- The heart rate goes up 10 seconds after each sleep bruxing event, indicative of stress activation [12]
- Blood pressure surges 20 to 25 percent with sleep bruxing. [13]
- Sleep bruxing aggravates painless periodontal disease, and periodontal inflammation has been linked to heart disease. [14, 15]

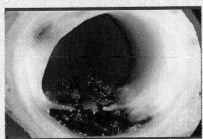

Bacteria DNA is 16 X higher in coronary thrombi than in blood samples
Pessi, et al, *Circulation*. 2013;127:1219-1228.

- 78.2% of thrombi w/ bacterial DNA, most Strep. Viridans

- 34.7% w/ perio. pathogens

- Periodontal and root canal infection can mean 13.2 X risk for heart attack

- "Dental infection and oral bacteria, especially viridans streptococci, may be associated with the development of acute coronary thrombosis."

Heart Attack:
Blood clot inside
ruptured coronary artery
Image courtesy of
Amy Doneen, R.N. and Brad Bale, M.D.

- A study in the Archives of Oral Biology found that sleep bruxing was present in 54 percent of mild OSA patients and 40 percent of moderate OSA patients. [16]

- 25 percent of patients with sleep apnea had sleep bruxing. [17]

- Teeth grinders are 80% more likely to self-report as having sleep apnea. [18]

- Teeth grinding is connected to airway obstruction because sleep bruxing can be eliminated using CPAP, or continuous positive airway pressure. [19]

In light of such evidence, teeth grinding may in fact be an early indicator of OSA.

Teeth Grinding: An Early Indicator of Sleep Apnea?

Teeth grinding is readily recognized in dental offices. With proper training, all health professionals and even most patients can recognize it. With proper training in providing Holistic Mouth

Checkups, dentists can be a valuable resource in early recognition of OSA risks to both teeth and hearts.

Consider J.J., whose wife expressed worry about him when she came in for a regular checkup and cleaning for herself. She said her 33-year old husband was grinding his teeth while sleeping. He snored, snorted, and gasped during sleep, she said, and woke up feeling tired every day. Sleepiness through the day was a problem, as well. Those last three symptoms are recognized signs of OSA, which accounts for 50 percent of high blood pressure cases, 30 percent of heart attacks, 60 percent of strokes, and 25 percent of heart failures. [20]

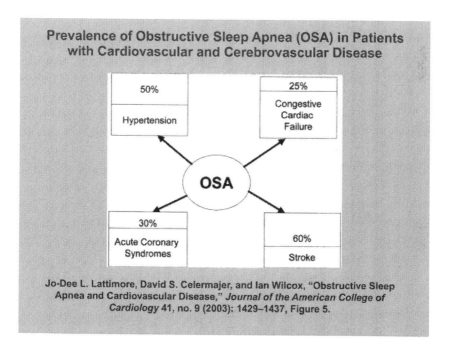

Prevalence of Obstructive Sleep Apnea (OSA) in Patients with Cardiovascular and Cerebrovascular Disease

Jo-Dee L. Lattimore, David S. Celermajer, and Ian Wilcox, "Obstructive Sleep Apnea and Cardiovascular Disease," *Journal of the American College of Cardiology* 41, no. 9 (2003): 1429–1437, Figure 5.

With his probable sleep apnea left unrecognized and untreated, J.J. may very well end up like S.G. in a decade or two. And in my experience, J.J. is hardly an exception.

From OSA to Heart Disease and Costly MACCEs

Major adverse coronary and cerebrovascular events (MACCEs) are among the most costly treatments driving up health care costs. They are also almost entirely preventable.

MACCEs are end results of a domino effect that starts with an impaired mouth, the tongue acting like a six-foot tiger in a three-foot cage. A study from Japan reported, "As compared with normal subjects, SDB [sleep disordered breathing] patients demonstrated receded mandibles and long lower faces with downward mandible development." [21] These are hallmarks of an impaired mouth.

The same study concluded that "obesity and craniofacial abnormalities contribute synergistically to increases in collapsibility of the passive pharyngeal airway in patients with SDB." This means a double chin should be taken seriously as a contributor to sleep apnea.

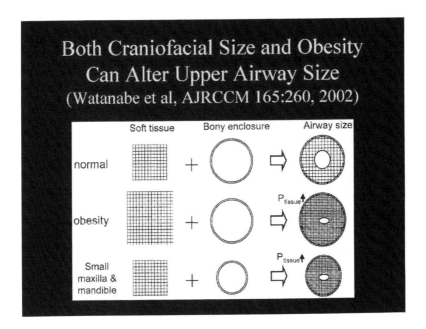

Other research agrees. For instance, one study published in the *New England Journal of Medicine* found that "snorers with and without sleep apnea have smaller pharyngeal [throat] cross-sectional areas than non-snorers," [22] This sets the body up for bankruptcy from an oxygen deficit night after night, which explains S.G.'s heart attack in the morning.

A 2014 study out of Singapore analyzed patients treated for acute coronary syndrome (ACS), which involves chest pain, jaw pain, arm numbness, and other symptoms stemming from a heart attack (blocked coronary artery). The researchers found that 35.3% of those treated for heart attack symptoms had at least moderate OSA. Two years later, patients in the OSA group had a 34.9% incidence of MACCEs compared with 5.1% for the non-OSA group. [23]

Translation: One out of three patients with heart attack symptoms had moderate to severe OSA, and those with OSA were about 7 times more likely to have a second heart attack, stroke, or heart failure compared with those without OSA.

Clearly, left unrecognized and untreated, OSA can kill, and often without warning. Dental offices certified to provide Holistic Mouth Checkups can offer an efficient way to identify OSA risks early in health's downhill slide toward sleep apnea.

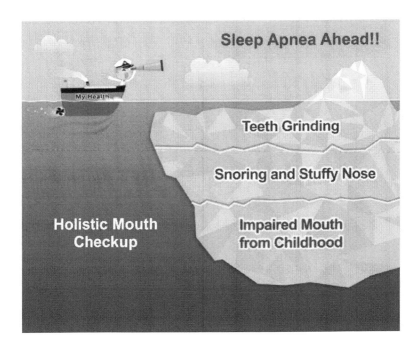

Update on S.G.

After many in-office consultation and on-line Q&As regarding his sleep test and pinched airway, S.G. decided not to start oral appliance therapy or CPAP because he felt he could not be compliant with either. Instead, he promised his wife he'd lose weight with diet and exercise. To his credit, S.G. has lost 30 pounds. But he still has not been regular with his dental checkup and cleanings.

This is human nature showing up in healthcare.

Holistic Mouth Nuggets

- High blood pressure can come from not only bad diet or emotional stress, but also sleep apnea and teeth grinding. Early diagnosis of sleep bruxing can save not only teeth but possibly the heart of a family's main wage earner.

- Double chin should be taken seriously as a surface sign of possible airway deficiency and contributor to sleep apnea, so should teeth grinding and its common complications such as chipped teeth, cracked roots, and failed root-canaled teeth — see chapter 11 next.

- Teeth grinding is readily recognized in dental offices. Non-dental health professionals certified as Holistic Mouth Consultants can be a valuable in the proactive management of OSA risks to save teeth and hearts.

Chapter 11

Dental Angina – Successful WholeHealth Rescue of Qualified Toothaches

Chronically ill patients need an informed dentist more than a medical doctor.

– Jerry Tennant, MD, author of *Healing Is Voltage*

What's bad for the heart is also bad for the tooth, and vice versa. That's a WholeHealth principle. The "nerve" inside a tooth is just as susceptible to oxygen deprivation as the coronary artery. If reduced blood flow can cause heart attack, can the same cause a tooth to ache?

Yes, and knowing this may just help many teeth from avoidable root-canal treatment. It is not uncommon for patients to have sensitivity and pain after "successful" dental treatment, where the dental work looks fine but the tooth just does not feel right. Sometimes, root-canal therapy may well be indicated, but too often, it is suggested for lack of a better "solution" to stop the lingering symptom(s).

Your actions as owner-operator of your mouth can lead to either happy endings – "The problem is solved and will never come back!" – or serious consequences, such as one dental trouble after another. Now let's see a new WholeHealth concept and Holistic Mouth Solutions™ can stop or reverse toothaches without root-canaled treatments — dental angina.

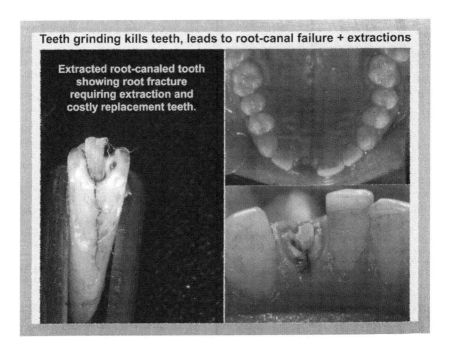

Teeth grinding kills teeth, leads to root-canal failure + extractions

Extracted root-canaled tooth showing root fracture requiring extraction and costly replacement teeth.

Angina: From Heart to Teeth

Dental angina is my term for early-stage toothache and dental sensitivity in the absence of cavities from reduced blood flow to a tooth, as in heart angina.

"Angina" notes the Mayo Clinic, "is a term used for chest pain caused by reduced blood flow to the heart muscle... Angina is typically described as squeezing, pressure, heaviness, tightness or pain in your chest." [1]

Airway obstruction during sleep is a known contributor to cardiac angina. [2, 3] One study suggests that "the high cardiovascular mortality rate reported in OSAS [obstructive sleep apnea syndrome] might not necessarily relate to underlying coronary artery disease." [4] In other words, there's more than cholesterol, salt and sugar in the mix — sleep apnea alone can kill.

Let's use a fist clench to experience an episode of reduced flow flow. If you're in good health – no history of heart angina, diabetes, or other risky medical condition – you can get an idea of what angina is like by making a fist and clenching it hard until your knuckles are white. Hold it for 11 seconds, then release.

Does it feel better to let go? What if release never comes?

If reduced blood flow in the heart causes chest pain, then the same can happen to a tooth's "nerve" (dental pulp) to cause toothache — especially the reduced blood flow is already low in oxygen from airway obstruction, and with jaw clenching na teeth grinding.

Now clench your jaws and squeeze your teeth for 11 seconds – but ONLY if your teeth and overall health are in good shape. Your teeth have just experienced an episode of sleep apnea with oxygen deprivation.

What if that clenching goes on all night long, every night, for years? That'd set up that pattern of one root-canal after another or extraction from cracked tooth. Many patients and their dentists are a risk of being surprised and frustrated by not knowing this, as the case of C.B. will show just ahead.

In my opinion, teeth are far more susceptible to angina because its blood pipeline is nearly 4 times smaller than a coronary artery. [5, 6] This explains why heart attack happens mostly in the second half of life, while non-cavity toothaches and dental sensitivities can take place at an earlier age.

As in heart angina, dental angina can come from atherosclerosis and chronic oxygen deficiency from airway obstruction. In addition, the dental pulp often suffers additional stress of jaw clenching, and teeth grinding. Lastly, the death of the dental pulp is accelerated once inflammation starts to build pressure inside the unyielding pulp chamber.

Imagine a garden hose with water running through it. Step on it, and the nozzle end dries up — simulating the jaw clenching and teeth grinding. Lift the squeeze, and the flow is restored — therein lies a simple solution.

If blood flow to the tooth is restored soon enough, dental angina should subside and the toothache should fade naturally. If not, death of the dental pulp will demand either an extraction or root-canal treatment. It's hardly rocket science, more like common sense.

This understanding of dental angina offers a WholeHealth solution for reversing them — by opening up the airway, relieving the jaw clenching, and soothing the trigger points.

Non-tooth Sources of Dental Angina

Besides jaw clenching, teeth grinding, and sleep apnea, dental angina may have more feeder sources:

- Diet and dental hygiene: 3 species of periodontal bacteria are found in heart attack clots in a 2012 study from Tokyo Dental College. "This raises the possibility that such bacteria are latently present in plaque and also suggests that these bacteria might have a role in plaque inflammation and instability." [7]

- Trigger Points: Symptoms are reactions to some cause, and the pain site can and often is apart from its source — see chapter 8. "A myofascial trigger point is a small, hypersensitive area within a that band of skeletal muscle." [8] "The most common neuromuscular trigger areas occur in the superior trapezius and sternocleidomastoid [muscles]." [9]

- Loss of enamel protection exposing the sensitive dentin and the pulp can come from cavities, drilling involved in dental work, or other causes.

Knowing as many of the non-dental causes and treating them accordingly may help resolve persistent pains and nagging sensitivity.

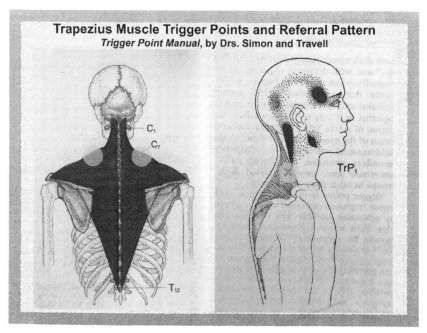

Image source above: Trigger Point Manual [10]
Image sources below: Neuromuscular Dentistry,
by Dr. Robert Jenkelson, DDS [11]

SCM Muscle Trigger Points
Refers to Ears, TMJ, Forehead, Mid-face

* Sterno-Cleido-Mastoid muscles: rope-shaped from back of ears to clavicle and top of breast bone

* Function: to turn head

* Very common with whiplash and impact trauma with head jerk

* SCM trigger points can come from car or bite accidents, poor head posture and/or computer monitor position

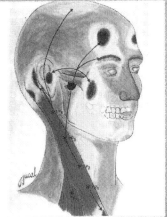

© Dr. Felix Liao, DDS   Image courtesy of Robert Jenkelson, DDS

Masseter Muscle Trigger Points
Refers to Upper and Lower Molars

* Masseter: jaw-clenching muscles in front of both ears

* Trigger points refer pain and tenderness to molars

* Very common pattern

* Masseter trigger points origin: teeth grinding, and/or narrow airway, and Trapezius muscle

* Trapezius trigger points from poor head posture

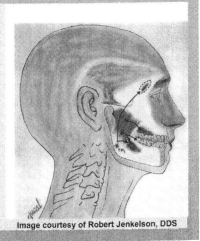

© Dr. Felix Liao, DDS   Image courtesy of Robert Jenkelson, DDS

In the absence of cavities or exposed dentin, it seems plausible to me that improving the link of sleep-airway-mouth on the one hand, and defusing trigger points on the other, have the potential to reduce dental sensitivities and reverse toothaches.

The two cases presented below highlight the difference between conventional and WholeHealth treatment of dental angina. Both patients – 56-year old CB and 41-year old BK – had regular cleanings with their respective dentists and came with excellent oral hygiene.

Pain Persists After Root-Canal Treatment and Extractions

C.B. came to me complaining of pain that began after a crown had been placed for a cracked molar (tooth #30). The pain had persisted despite root-canal treatment by an excellent root-canal specialist. So tooth #30 was extracted. In the meantime, the same pain happened to the same molar (#19) on her other side. C.B. liked her dentist, so she let him repeat the same treatment for #19. Pain persisted again in #19.

Both teeth were eventually extracted, but still her pain persisted. Chair Side Investigation (CSI) on her history and in her mouth showed:

1. Tooth #30 cracked while chewing 2 years ago. A new crown resulted in lots of pain.
2. Root-canal treatment on #30 by specialist resulted in 50% reduction of pain.
3. Pain in tooth #19 began shortly after root-canal treatment on #30. Pain in #19 led to another root-canal treatment.
4. Pain in both teeth remains unchanged 2 months after they were both extracted.
5. Presenting symptoms included snoring, teeth grinding, clicking jaw joints, morning headaches and sore jaws, neck and shoulder pain, weight gain and abdominal obesity, daytime sleepiness and fatigue, senile memory/ADHD, acid reflux, depression, anxiety, grouchiness, and "lots of tension in chest".

These are not typically tooth doctor's concerns, but they are significant clues to a doctor of Holistic Mouth.

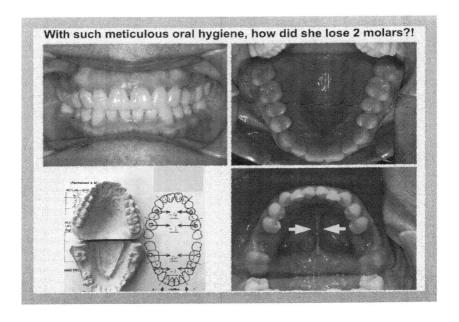

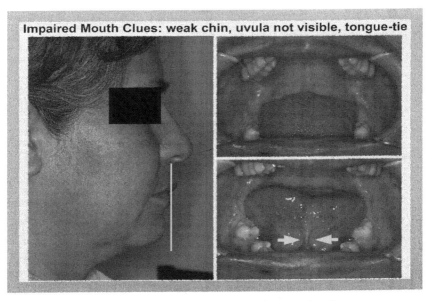

Yellow plumb line suggests Liao's Sign implicating
Impaired Mouth and Pinched Airway

Serious risks and consequences can come from staying inside the traditional dental box, using only panoramic x-rays and study casts to determine irreversible treatment. In C.B.'s case, two teeth were treated and lost without considering the possible causes. Implants are next, and it's costly to both C.B. and her dentist who has offered to credit her for the money she paid for the failed root-canals and subsequent oral surgery.

Better outcomes require different thinking. In my opinion, CB's toothaches likely came from dental angina and possibly trigger points in her masseter muscles, neither of which were addressed by her previous "in-the-dental-box" treatment.

CB's cone beam CT imaging showed a significantly narrow airway with a high risk of collapse during sleep.

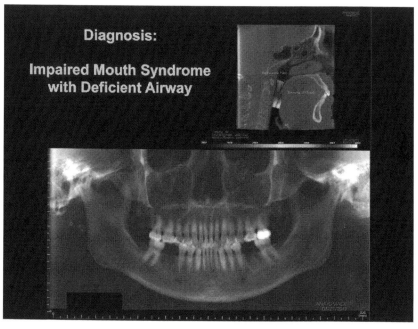

Consider the airway and its effect on the dental pulp before starting restorative or endodontic treatment.

Dental angina is the oral version of a heart attack in a tooth's "nerve", and the pain can come from chronic oxygen starvation. What if we were to relieve the oxygen deficiency and treat the trigger points? Now let's see B.K.'s story.

Dental Treatment Outcome from Adopting the WholeHealth View

B.K. was desperate to avoid root-canal treatment on an increasingly painful tooth after a new crown had been placed on a molar (tooth#18) by a highly respected biological dentist. Adjusting its bite did not relieve her pain. At the time, she came to see me, she was wearing a TMJ splint similar to a sports mouth guard 24 hours a day.

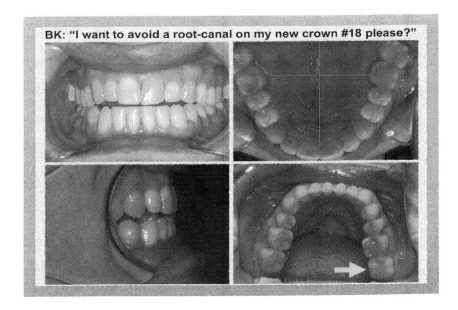

Her presenting complaints included:

- Pain in the lower left jaw ("I have not chewed on left side for over a year.")
- A new crown #18 tender to bite.
- Left TMJ clicks for which she was wearing a dentist-made appliance full-time.
- Recent neck crackling and chronic shoulder pain.
- Multiple chemical sensitivity.

"All my pains and maladies are left-sided," BK added. This pattern is a big red flag in the WholeHealth view: putting a crown on her tooth #18 (lower left second molar) is risky, but this red flag is not seen in dentistry's silo.

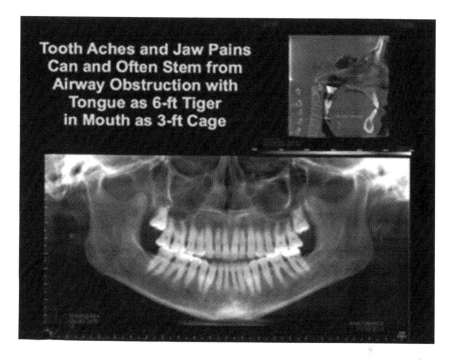

B.K.'s anterior open bite resulted from having a normal size-six tongue inside a size-three mouth. It told me that she was suffering from Impaired Mouth Syndrome undiagnosed.

Cephalometric analysis showed that she had an undiagnosed class III malocclusion. Her maxilla (upper jaw) was retruded, and both maxilla and mandible were entrapped. These combined to give her neck and shoulder pain. CBCT imaging also showed that her airway was 30 to 50% from low normal and that her cervical spinal segments were misaligned.

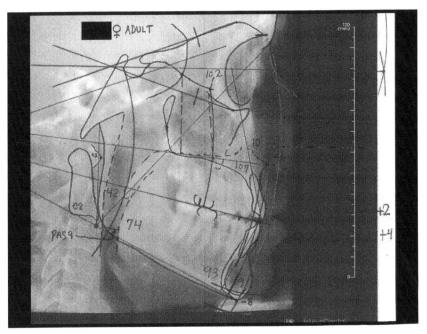

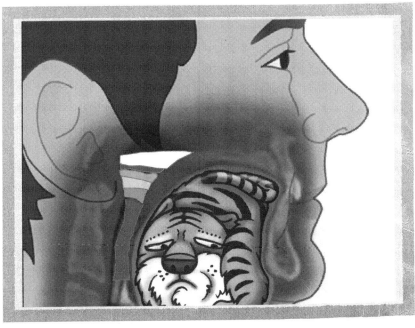

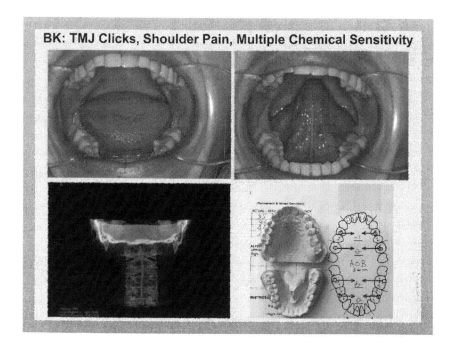

BK: TMJ Clicks, Shoulder Pain, Multiple Chemical Sensitivity

Seen in the WholeHealth light, B.K's pain after the new crown likely was the side effects of her pre-existing TMD, cranio-mandibular sacral asymmetry, and injuries. The solution wasn't to file down the crown or put her on anti-inflammatories or antibiotics. That's inside-the-dental-box thinking.

Instead, I directed her treatment toward opening the airway via oral expander appliance therapy. I also referred her for cranio-sacral therapy, breathing lessons, posture training, and acupuncture to defuse her trigger points.

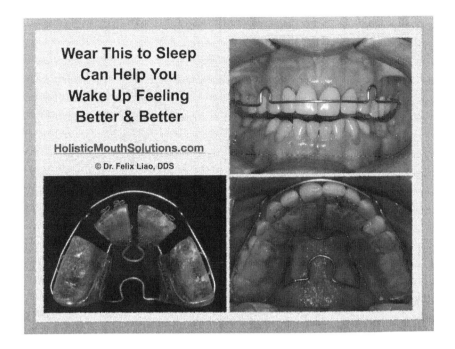

A Better Outcome with Holistic Mouth Solutions™

Ten months after starting her Holistic Mouth Solutions treatment, B.K. had not had root-canal treatment. "I wanted you to know how grateful I feel," she wrote to me.

> Your understanding of how the body works from a much larger WholeHealth perspective than any previous dentist seems to have saved me. Without your appliance in my mouth, I have jaw pain. With the appliance, there's no pain.

> Before I came to you, it was recommended that I either break and re-align my jaw with surgery or that I might have a jaw bone infection that would also require extensive surgery. The pain went away with the appliance, showing that it wasn't an infection issue. I also feel relief and have faith that the alignment work you're doing will save me from any surgery.

Still, she must remain vigilant. "Your toothache can come back if your trigger points or stress level come back above some invisible level," I reminded her. "The oral appliance starts the process of reducing your bad bite as a source, but YOU are responsible for the control of trigger points by staying physically relaxed and emotionally even-keeled. Call me right away if your stress exceeds your tooth's threshold."

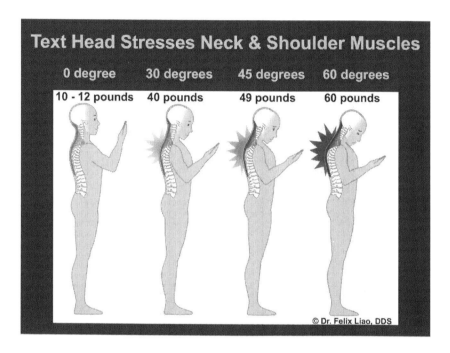

Timeliness by the Patient Makes Superior Doctor

Pain demands action, and sometimes you have no choice but to focus on putting out the fire. But do you really want to just treat the pain or to eliminate its cause? But that requires two things from you:

A. You have to do your part for your overall health with sleep, diet, exercise, dental hygiene, stress management;

B. You must act in time – within 24 to 48 hours of onset, not months later when you cannot stand the pain anymore.

The rest depends on whether your dentist is "in-the-box" or open to WholeHealth connections and solutions.

Holistic Mouth Nuggets:

- In the absence of cavities and gum disease, dental angina should be considered as a possible cause of dental sensitivity and toothaches. Before rushing to root-canal treatment, identifying – or ruling out – jaw clenching and sleep bruxing can lead to better outcomes.

- What's bad for the heart is also bad for the tooth. WholeHealth-oriented Holistic Mouth Solutions™ can remove trigger points and airway obstruction can be helpful to keep dental angina at bay and some (not all) sensitive teeth from root-canal treatment.

- To avoid dental angina, reduce inflammation with low-carb diet, identify and de-escalate trigger points, control their perpetuating factors, and consider a customized oral appliance to address your jaw clenching and teeth grinding.

Chapter 12

The Tyranny of Malocclusion - Pain, Fatigue, and Many Nasty Side Effects

If your (chiropractic) adjustments are not holding, consider seeing a dentist who knows how to treat malocclusion.

– Dr. Yvonne Petrie, Doctor of Chiropractics

Neck aches and shoulder pain are among the most frequent complaints to massage therapists, chiropractors, and to me when new patients come to see me. Why? More importantly, why do the aches and pains keep coming back? Patients often shake their heads and shrug their shoulders when I ask.

Symptom management may feel good for a day or two, then the old pattern comes back. That is the problem with fragmented care. Worse yet, with chronic pain comes fatigue, depression, and adrenal exhaustion. Until the faucet is turned off, water will keep overflowing onto the bathroom floor.

In many cases, the culprit is malocclusion (bad bite), another cardinal feature of an Impaired Mouth that interferes with alignment, breathing circulation, digestion, energy, and sleep.

In WholeHealth, malocclusion is more than just crowded, crooked teeth in need of a smile makeover. Malocclusion is the absence of alignment of the cranium, spine, jaws, and teeth, and a much-neglected source of health troubles.

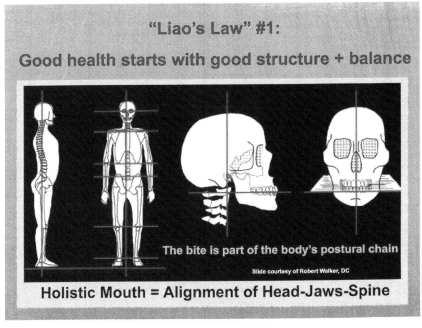

Graphic illustration provided by Robert Walker, D.C.

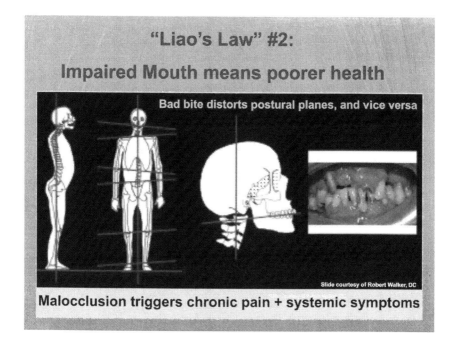

Alignment: Why Good Health Starts with Good Structure

The body's postural chain from head to feet is organized to resist gravity and provide mobility. Since gravity never stops pulling us toward the grave, misalignment means health troubles: pain, fatigue, disease, dysfunction, less energy, lower life quality, and higher healthcare costs.

Alignment here means a level and square frame to provide airway, blood flow, and nerve supplies for superior muscle performance in sports and in daily living. Alignment is the Law of Form and Function at work:

good form = good function = good health

Alignment is the first requirement for health, because it provides the proper form for efficient function. Imagine driving a race car with a bent frame. The same holds for going through life with misalignment. This is why so many patients get unexpectedly better when malocclusion is properly treated.

Alignment of the head, jaws, bite, and spine is the first criterion for Holistic Mouth. A good dental bite follows and supports orthopedic alignment so you don't have to run to the chiropractor or massage therapist as often.

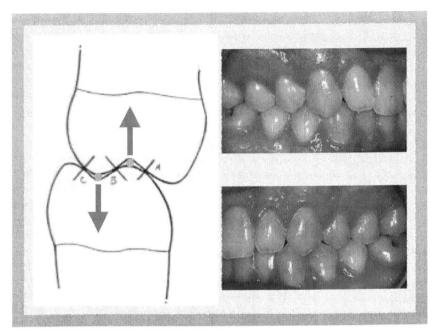

*Good occlusion has stable peak-to-valley fit that
directs forces along the long axes of teeth
(green arrows).*

Malocclusion Signs and Symptoms

Crowded, crooked teeth are just one feature of malocclusion. Here are more common tell-tale signs:

- A deep overbite, with the edge of the upper front teeth overlapping the lower by more than 2 mm.

- A cross bite, in which one or more lower teeth is closer to the cheek or tongue than the corresponding teeth above it.

- An open bite, in which the upper and lower teeth fail to make contact when the jaws come together.

- An excessive overjet, with the lower front teeth more than 2 mm behind the upper front teeth (Class II, often appears as weak chin)

- An excessive overjet with the lower front teeth ahead of the upper front teeth (Class III, often appears as bulbous chin and weak midface).

- An uneven bite. The upper and lower front teeth may meet at a slant, with one side higher than the other – a recipe for headache, neck pain, and dental troubles. Or the lower front teeth may meet higher than the back teeth. Or one side of the upper teeth may be higher than the other. In these cases, the TMJ often pays the price, with clicking, popping, locking, bruxing, muscle aches, and trigger points being common.

- Matching wear and tear on teeth on the cutting edges of the front and side teeth from teeth grinding, which if excessive can lead to sensitivity to cold and sweets.

- Abfractions: notches on the exposed roots at the gums lines, usually on the lip-side of teeth. These abfractions are often associated with teeth grinding. They can be very sensitive to cold and brushing.

- Excessive bony outgrowths on jaws called torus (the plural is tori) that come from long-term jaw clenching or teeth grinding.

- TMJ (temporomandibular joint) issues, including clicking, popping, and locking jaw joints, or aches and pains in head, face, teeth, jaws, neck, shoulders, etc. — see chapter 13 next.

Medical-Dental Consequences of Malocclusion

Malocclusion is a big bother to the brain and the whole body. This was well documented by Dr. Aelred Fonder in the 1970s. [4] Dr. Fonder's observations were confirmed by a revealing 1989 study out of Japan's Kyoto University of Medicine. I am grateful to Dr. Ara Elmajian, a great biological dentist and friend, who brought it to my attention.

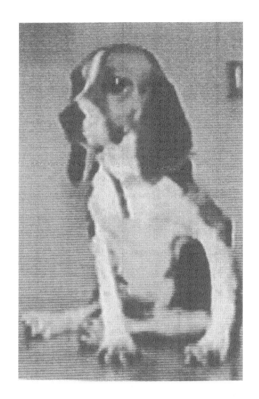

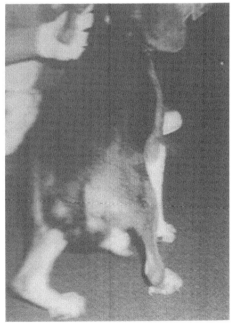

For this study, malocclusion was experimentally induced in beagles by cutting their back teeth short on the right side so they did not meet. The dogs were then observed for a year. Within a week, their lower midlines had shifted to the right. There was tearing and salivation. There was a loss of hair luster. Two of the three dogs showed weakness in their left hind legs and walked lame. Yet blood tests, weight, and stool samples showed no abnormal changes – a reminder that routine medical tests cannot disclose these types of postural, gait, and dental-facial symptoms. [1]

The takeaway: bad bite means bad posture, and bad posture implicates bad bite.

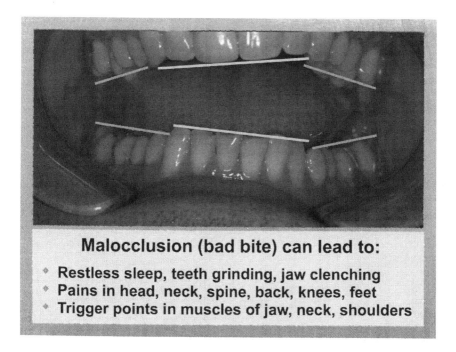

Malocclusion (bad bite) can lead to:

* Restless sleep, teeth grinding, jaw clenching
* Pains in head, neck, spine, back, knees, feet
* Trigger points in muscles of jaw, neck, shoulders

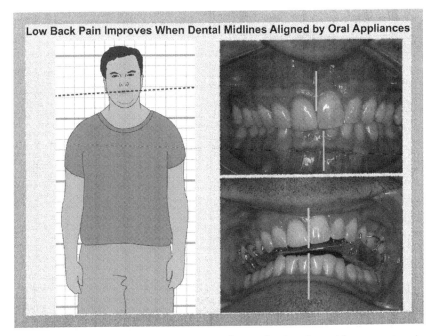

Oral appliance took away this patient's chronic back pain and he won a tennis tournament in his club without back and knee braces a few months later.

Malocclusion: Wide Spread and Under-treated

Only 35% of adults have well-aligned mandibular incisors. Data from the third National Health and Nutrition Examination Survey (NHANES III) provide a clear picture of malocclusion in the US population:

- Noticeable incisor irregularity occurs in most people, regardless of race/ethnicity. The irregularity is severe enough in 15% that both social acceptability and function could be affected, and major arch expansion or extraction of some teeth would be required for correction.

- About 20% have deviations from the ideal bite relationship. In 2%, these are severe enough to be disfiguring and are at the limit for orthodontic correction.

- More than half – 57 to 59% - of those surveyed needed at least some need for orthodontic treatment. [2]

In hospitals and doctors' offices, malocclusion is under-recognized. In dental offices, malocclusion is under-treated. That's how Impaired Mouth Syndrome goes unrecognized.

In my experience, it is the neck and head that invariably pay the price of pain and fatigue in the presence of malocclusion. That pain is eased or resolved, patients frequently report, with oral appliance therapy.

Malocclusion Treatment

Orthodontics is one way to treat malocclusion. You also see restorative and prosthodontic procedures used, or various combinations of all of these. (Prosthodontics is the dental specialty that deals with replacing natural teeth with man-made teeth with bridgework, dentures, and implants.)

Epigenetic orthopedics is another way to treat malocclusion – that is, the use of oral appliances such as expanders and oral-face masks to change jaw to jaw or jaw to skull relationships.

In most American dental offices today, malocclusion is more managed than treated. Symptoms are fixed – teeth straightened cosmetically, sensitive teeth repaired with restorations, toothaches addressed with root-canals – but their structural causes remain unaddressed.

Orthodontic correction lines up teeth like boxcars on a railroad, while epigenetic orthopedics corrects the railroad bed. Treating malocclusion in WholeHealth means correcting the bad bite so it is no longer a stressor to whole body health.

The Case of Dr. P.Y.

"I've had neck pain for ages," said Dr. P.Y., a chiropractic doctor who came to see me. "And I've been grinding my teeth for as long as I can remember. My neck pain gets relief from chiropractic adjustment, but it comes back the next day."

Dr. P.Y.'s complaint is typical. Neck and shoulder pain ranks number one in most massage therapists' offices. When it keeps coming back, remember malocclusion.

A customized oral appliance can release the head-jaw-neck-shoulder muscle pain naturally. In Dr. P.Y.'s case, the oral appliance also served as a sleep aid, TMJ appliance, and palatal expander. Three weeks after starting therapy, she reported that her pain "goes away within a half hour of putting on my bite correction appliance, and I feel refreshed in the morning after sleeping with my appliance overnight."

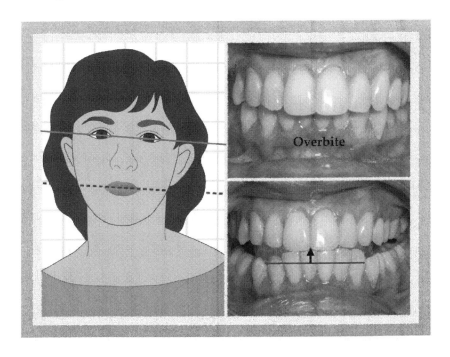

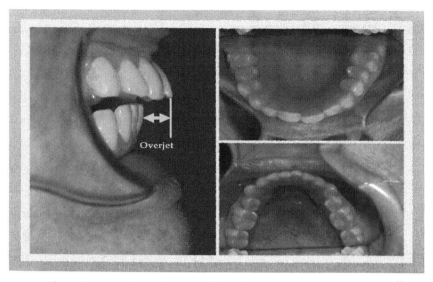

Above: impaired mouth case with head tilt, malocclusion featuring moderate overjet, open bite and deficient jaws. Below: neck pain goes away after lower jaw is freed from its entrapment with oral appliances.

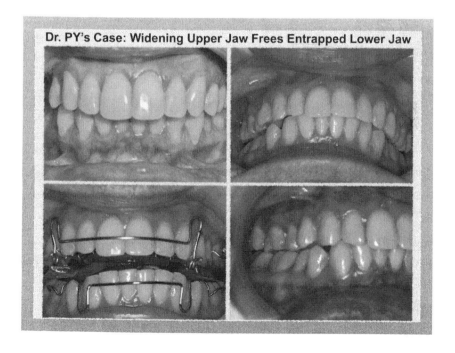

Dr. P.Y.'s symptoms stemmed from skeletal malocclusion, or orthopedic misalignment of the jaws in relation to each other (under- or over-bite), or of the jaw(s) in relationship to the skull (weak chin, or upper jaw retrusion resulting in flat cheek bones). Correctly diagnosing and treating both the skeletal *and* dental malocclusion can make associated headaches and neck-back pains go away naturally.

Dr. P.Y. is an exceptional doctor in that she knows and believes in the need to integrate chiropractic with Holistic Mouth as a natural solution. In my experience, chiropractic doctors are among the more aware non-dental health professionals.

Malocclusion in The WholeHealth Context

The bite is connected to head, neck, and back, and thus also airway and sleep. Too many patients suffer the consequences because too many healthcare professionals remain unaware of this point.

Malocclusion can trigger pain to the head, neck, and whole body. It is also a perpetuating stressor. "Dental malocclusion, bruxism, and emotional tension can interact to overload the masticatory and neck muscles perpetuating their TPs [trigger points] and producing much of the head and face pain of the myofascial pain dysfunction syndrome." [3]

Interestingly, if a patient feels no pain or fatigue in the presence of malocclusion and a pinched airway, it may be the effect of cortisol. That hormone helps us cope with chronic stress, like a good soldier who carries on the fight without whining, despite being exhausted and wounded. But this comes at a high health cost later, as Dr. Robert Sapolsky explains so well in *Why Zebras Don't Get Ulcers* – a book I recommend highly. [4]

In my experience, adrenal support is a frequent need among sleep apnea patients due to nightly struggle to stay alive for years. Besides mopping up the symptoms of adrenal exhaustion, attending to predisposing factors is important to "turn off the faucet". Predisposing factors frequently include

- Structural and postural inadequacies and muscle tension.
- Nutritional deficiencies.
- Metabolic and endocrine (hormonal) deficiencies.
- Depression, anxiety, tension, and other psychological factors.
- Chronic infections and infestations.
- Impaired sleep, allergies/runny-/stuffy nose, pinched nerves.

According to the authors of the *Myofascial Pain Dysfunction Trigger Point Manual,* paying attention to these predisposing factors "in patients with chronic myofascial pain… often spells the difference between successful and failed therapy." [5]

The association between gum inflammation and heart disease is becoming better known in the integrative medical community. The same needs to happen with malocclusion and Impaired Mouth Syndrome. Failure to recognize malocclusion results in far too many dental-medical-mood symptoms and much higher expenses on managing pain, dysfunction, and disease, as we shall see next.

Holistic Mouth Nuggets:

- Alignment is a much-overlooked foundation for natural health and wellness. Misalignment means poorer health, and vice versa.
- Malocclusion is a reflection of cranial-facial-jaw misalignment underneath. A simple oral appliance can often be useful in uncomplicated cases, i.e. without trauma or injury or prior surgery.
- Chronic pain, fatigue, and other Impaired Mouth Syndrome symptoms are simply downstream consequences of skeletal malocclusion left untreated. Conversely, many symptoms either improve or resolve naturally when skeletal malocclusion is successfully corrected.

- Malocclusion is a much-overlooked trigger and perpetuating factor in chronic pain and fatigue that can undermine nutrition, medication, fitness, lifestyle, and stress management.

Chapter 13

"Thank you for giving my wife back to me, Doc." — A Primer on TMJ Pain & Dysfunction

The triad of TMJD, sleep disordered breathing, and malocclusion may co-present as undiagnosed cranio-facial development.

– Dr. G. Dave Singh [1]

Do your jaw joints click, pop, or lock? Does your lower jaw open and close in a smooth straight line or zig-zag? Do you have trouble opening wide enough to bite into a piled-high sandwich or for dental work? Do you have aches and pains in your head, face, neck, or shoulders? These are some of the common signs of temporomandibular joint dysfunction (TMJD, often shortened to TMJ or TMD).

TMJ is where the mandible (lower jaw) is attached to the back half of the cranium — that "igloo" made of eight bones to house the brain. What if it were your hip or knee joint clicking or jerking with each step you took, or your elbow and wrist with each hand movement? Most people would run to the orthopedist right away, yet many people live with TMJ dysfunction, unaware of its WholeHealth consequences.

In WholeHealth, TMJ pain and dysfunction reflect misalignment in the craniofacial bones, which have their own postural chain just like spinal segments. So treatment prescribed in Holistic Mouth Solutions™ is not directed solely at the jaw joint or the jaw muscles, but at redeveloping the jaws so they align with the cranium and the neck spine to provide a sound structure to the body's Command & Control center.

You can take out your contact lenses or take off overly tight clothing when you get home, but you can't take off your malocclusion or TMJs. TMJs is a frequent aspect of malocclusion, and they do not have to hurt to hurt your whole body health. Let's see why.

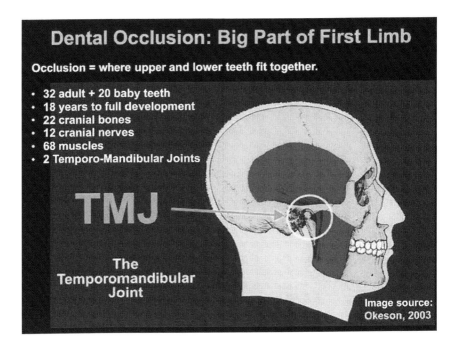

196

Assessing and Knowing Your TMJ

Clicking jaw joints mean they are jammed into the skull bone(s) housing your ears whenever you bite together. The sound comes from the cartilage slipping off from between the ball-and-socket of the jaw joints where it belongs. "The clicking and popping…is often of neuro-muscular etiology." [2]

Dental occlusion (the bite) is where and how upper and lower teeth come together to chew and swallow, a vital function that we take for granted. Upper teeth are rooted in the maxilla which is attached the front half of the head, and lower teeth in the mandible which is attached to the back half of the head. With proper form and alignment in both jaws, teeth can bite together in harmony which provides the head with "neurological peace".

With deficient form and misalignment in either jaw resulting in bad bite, TMJ pays the price of being compressed, and the whole body suffers the tyranny of malocclusion. You can assess your TMJs very easily two ways:

1. **Three finger test**. Open as wide as you can without pain and see if you can fit the middle three fingers of your hand between your teeth. If you cannot do this, it suggests a limited range of motion in your TMJs. Naturally, that comes with consequences.
2. **The pinkie test**. Just place your pinkie fingers in your ear openings, finger pads forward, then open and close your mouth. If you can feel pushback by your jaw joints when you close or if you hear clicking, you likely have TMJ dysfunction.

Thus, your TMJ clicks and your jaw's range of motion reflect the size and position of your jaws. TMJ signs and symptoms, even the painless clicks, mean you do not have enough room in your head for all its components, and that is not good for sleep and health. Knowing this can head off bigger oral-systemic health troubles ahead.

Meet Your Jaws Joints and Jaw Muscles

Your jaw joints move in finely tuned coordination to eat, drink, swallow, smile, speak, and express feelings. This smooth coordination requires lots of precise neurological teamwork in the brain. Indeed, the jaws and teeth are supplied by the largest of twelve cranial nerves.

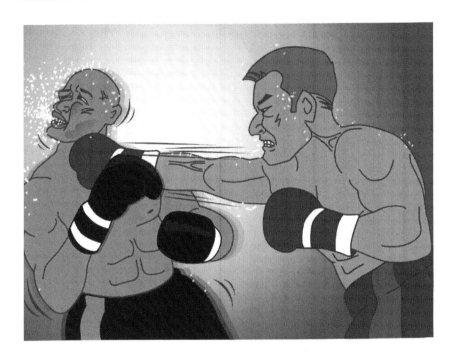

In boxing, the sweet spots for a knockout punch are the temples, jaws, and chin. These "lights out" areas remind us that the jaws serve as the brain's shock absorbers and circuit breakers. No anatomy lesson is needed to see that the jaws are directly wired to the body's command and control center, the brain.

Outside the boxing ring, in daily life, the TMJs and jaw muscles bear the brunt of mental-emotional stress and swallowed feelings. To locate your jaw muscles, put the palms of your hands on your cheeks, with the webs of your thumbs around your earlobes and the tips of your index and middle fingers at your temples. Now clench your jaw and grind your teeth. Those jaw muscles bulging under your palms are the masseters. The ones under your fingertips are the temporalis muscles. These muscles are frequent sources of trigger points that contribute to toothaches.

"Strong muscle contractions can cut off capillary flow and deplete the nutrient supply (oxygen) to the muscles, leading to "almost complete muscle fatigue within approximately 1 minute." [3]

The TMJs are unique in that the mandible is the only bone with joints on both sides of your body. That means an action like chewing requires lots of coordination from many neurons. Indeed, the TMJs are innervated by the largest of the Cranial Nerves supplying the head. Dr. Dietrich Klinghardt offers some fascinating insights to the dynamics of malocclusion.

> Chewing is the primary mechanism necessary for our survival. It is my firm opinion that the entire human organism is designed around the chewing mechanism and not around the brain, and not around walking/locomotion, as many others think.

> If there is malocclusion, the entire organism will try immediately to adapt to this situation, so that food can be processed optimally. The cranium will distort in a way that will help the upper and lower teeth to approximate. This distortion will create distortion of entire cranial-sacral lining from upper neck and tail bone.

> If the distortion of the cranium is not enough to compensate for malocclusion and the orthopedic misalignment of the jaws, the cervical spine will start to compensate, resulting in distortion of the neck, upper back, and the should girdle in order to create asymmetric leverage for the muscles involved in the chewing mechanism.

> The above-named mechanisms are responsible for such varied symptoms as depression (compromised of blood flow to certain areas of brain), loss of concentration, insomnia,

headaches, neck pain, low back pain – all caused by TMJ Dysfunction.

Keeping Dr. Klinghardt's view of TMJ and malocclusion in mind can help WholeHealth-minded professionals can better serve their patients, particularly if jaw retrusion is understood as a concept and diagnosed as a feature of Impaired Mouth.

Retruded TMJ Consequences

TMJ dysfunction happens when the mandible is trapped by the dental bite in a retruded position. Retrusion in the "3-foot cage" metaphor means deficient front-back length, while deep bite means low ceiling.

Retrusion is the opposite of protrusion. Retrusion jams the jaw joints into the temporal bone housing the ears, which are in charge not just of hearing but the sense of balance, as you will see in chapter 18.

In jaw development, the maxilla leads, and the mandible follows. Dr. Richard Beistle, an orthodontic instructor for United States Dental Institute, describes the maxilla as the shoe, and the mandible as the foot. This helps us understand what happens to the TMJs when the maxilla is undersized, or retruded.

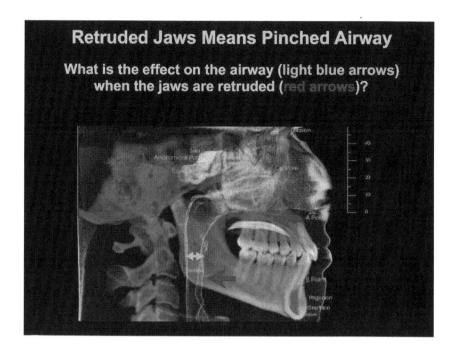

Retruded Jaws Means Pinched Airway

What is the effect on the airway (light blue arrows) when the jaws are retruded (red arrows)?

A retruded maxilla often causes the mandible to take up a retruded position and thereby drive the tongue further into the airway. A retruded maxilla means a flat cheek bones and sunken mid-face, and the chin often looks excessive as a result. A retruded mandible means weak chin, double chin, and frequently TMJ dysfunction.

A brilliant study out of Baylor University found that in rats, there was less genetic activity in a retruded TMJ and more in the the protruded joint. [4] This suggests that a retruded TMJ can block full genetic potential.

Conversely, freeing the mandible from its entrapment (retrusion) can bring on fuller genetic potential. That's quite a revelation to me. The big pearl: freeing the mandible from entrapment requires redevelopment of the maxilla. This explains why mandibular advancement appliances for sleep apnea have limited results.

The whole body benefits if we can decompress the TMJ from its retruded position. That's why facial radiance and upbeat mood are usually part of the outcome from implementing Holistic Mouth solutions. In summary, these are the more common factors that lead to TMJ dysfunction:

- A retruded maxilla.
- A narrow maxilla.
- A retruded mandible.
- A deep overbite.
- Cranial asymmetry or imbalance.
- Trauma impacts. such as jaw injuries, chin smacks, or whiplash.

By addressing these and other perpetuating factors, we can turn an Impaired Mouth into a Holistic Mouth as part of an overall wellness program.

Tandem Treatment: WholeHealth Teamwork

A tandem bike is one bicycle with two wheels and seats for two riders. A tandem treatment is one treatment plan with two doctors on the same WholeHealth platform.

TMJ Dysfunction can and often does affect the Atlas-Axis joint where your head is mounted on the top of your spine. This is why neck and shoulder pain are regular features of TMJ dysfunction. It's also why tandem teamwork between healthcare professionals, body workers, and Holistic Mouth doctors is important.

The atlas-malocclusion link also explains why a correctly diagnosed and designed appliance can and often relieve neck-shoulder-back pain. There are two exceptions: (A) when the TMJs are too damaged, in which case surgery may be needed, or (B) a history of traumatic blows to the jaw (bar fights, bike handle bar, assaults, or whiplash from accidents) in which case tandeom treatment is mandatory to restore the hard and soft tissues back into alignment.

WholeHealth collaboration produces the best results. Team work among chiropractic, osteopathic, orthopedic, medical doctors, physical therapists, acupuncturists, athletic trainers, and Holistic Mouth doctors trained in airway redevelopment and oral appliances can solve many cases of chronic pain that prove resistant to standard piecemeal care.

In my practice, patients with Impaired Mouth patients starting oral appliance therapy are routinely referred for postural training and breathing lessons, oral-facial myofunctional and cranio-sacral therapy, chiropractic adjustments, physical and/or massage therapy, Traditional Chinese Medicine, and/or acupuncture, as needed.

The Case of T.M.

Twenty-year old T.M. was referred to me by his chiropractic doctor who was treating him for scoliosis. "I'm so tired —I can't hold down a job," he said, "and my family can't understand why." His presenting symptoms included:

- Chronic fatigue worsening recently.
- Very low stress tolerance and easily annoyed by noise.
- Snoring.
- Sore chewing muscles from clenching jaws during the day.
- Clicking and popping TMJs.

Significant aspects of his health history included a medical diagnosis of moderate obstructive sleep apnea (AHI = 19.8), military service, and braces in middle school. He admits to being over-thinking and worrying.

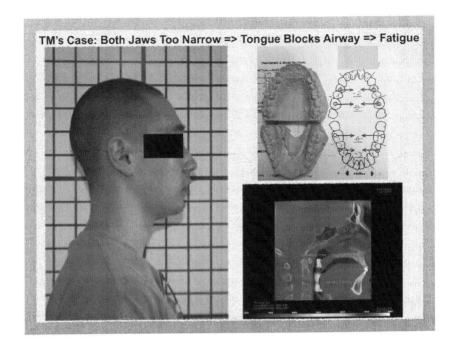

TM's Case: Both Jaws Too Narrow => Tongue Blocks Airway => Fatigue

My examination found a positive pinkie test, further suggesting TMJ dysfunction, and also saw that his lower jaw deviated to the right, likewise indicating problems is worse on his right TMJ. The logical recommendation was oral appliance therapy.

T.M. also showed signs of nasal congestion and habitual mouth breathing – situations best addressed through myofunctional therapy, Buteyko breathing exercises, using a Lip Trainer™ to strengthen the orofacial muscles, dietary changes, and referral to a WholeHealth acupuncturist for digestive support.

While undergoing treatment with me, he would continue seeing his chiropractor so his adjustments for scoliosis would be complemented with the oral appliance therapy. I call this "tandem treatment."

In T.M.'s case, having the bite on his oral appliance balanced after a chiropractic adjustment avoided the usual relapse that comes from ignoring the adverse influence of malocclusion driving the old pattern of misalignment. Kudos to his WholeHealth oriented chiropractic doctor.

How is T.M. after the tandem treatment? "My health is pretty good now," he says. "My sweating is down, I don't wake up to go to the bathroom, and my fatigue is down to 2 on a scale of 10. My TMJ pain is gone, and my scoliosis is better."

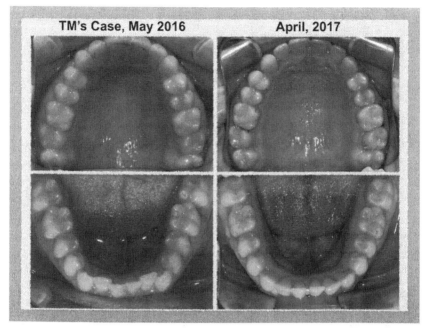

Above: note lower front teeth on lower right image
(after treatment) is no longer crowded

Below: changes in the airway after 9 months of sleeping with
upper and lower oral appliances + oral face mask.

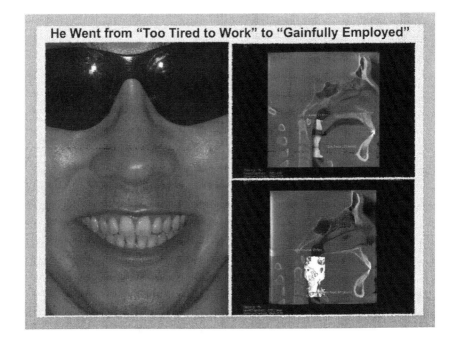

He Went from "Too Tired to Work" to "Gainfully Employed"

Misalignment Means TMJ-Neck-Back Pain

Pain and dysfunction show up when spinal vertebrae are out of alignment with each other. The same happens with craniofacial bones. Misalignment within the craniofacial skeleton can make life miserable, as the case of RK and others ahead will show.

Without turning this into an anatomy textbook, here's are some of the key TMJ connections to the whole body:

- The Trigeminal Nerve has branches that goes down to mid-neck, which explains why jaw and neck pain often run together, and why treating malocclusion and TMJ dysfunction often helps neck pain. "The dentist must be the primary diagnostician and therapist of those muscles and associated structures innervated by the trigeminal nerve... The ultimate objective of occlusal management is to provide an occlusal position most conducive to relaxation of the posturing muscles of the head and neck." [5]

- Malocclusion activates a wakefulness network of neurons called reticular activating system in the brain stem to increase insomnia and anxiety. "Excessive arousal in the reticular activating system can lead to heightened state of anxiety, fear, and uncertainty... Problem with insomnia are common in the TMJ/MSD (musculo-skeletal dysfunction, or bodily pain) patients." [6]

- The spine and the soft tissue fascia connect the TMJs to mid- and low back, which explains why treating malocclusion can help low back pain in many cases.

- Postural distortion and malocclusion are connected.

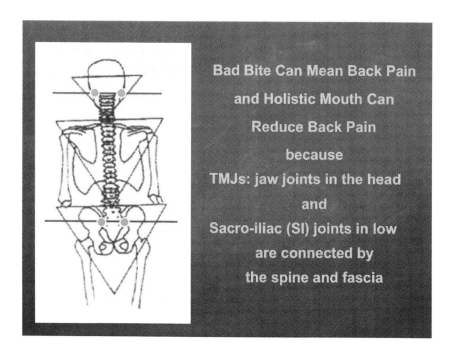

The intelligent design of the body places four sensors to sense structural alignment in four strategic spots: two in the low back called the *sacroiliac joints* (SIJ) and two in the jaw joints (TMJ). The two pairs are connected by the spine.

So, when the SI joints in the hips are off, the TMJ and the bite are out of alignment. This is frequently the case with mothers holding up kids on their hips. The reverse also matters in cases of pronated feet without sufficient arch support. Correct the postural alignment before doing any major dental work.

WholeHealth sees the body as one postural chain made up of head-neck-spine-legs and including the two jaws and the 32 adult teeth in peak-to-valley fit when they bite together. This fit can reinforce the entire postural chain or distort it with symptoms anywhere in the body. Understanding the relationships among the head, jaws, bite, and spine is important for effective treatment for many cases of nagging pain that keeps coming back.

Bad Back from Bad Bite?! The Case of RK

"You're saying my bad back can be connected to my bad bite?" said R.K. "I've never heard that."

R.K. was a part-time journalist who loved to eat heathy, work out, dance, and hike. She interviewed me three times because she could not believe that her back pain could be connected to her bite. "I've maxed out five chiropractors and osteopaths in five years. Now it hurts even to turn over in bed."

"It's simple to find out, without any side effects," I told her. "You can try wearing an oral appliance similar to a mouthpiece an athlete may wear. The difference is that this one allows your body to be free of the tyranny of your bad bite."

"I have no choice after the dinner party where I couldn't stand for more than fifteen minutes and had to sit like an old lady. No one sat down to talk to me all night long."

She finally started treatment after Thanksgiving weekend, on one condition: "I have had a hiking trip planned in February, and this had better work."

"The appliance will tell you within the first week if the arrow is pointing the right direction. But you need to combine oral appliance therapy with chiropractic/osteopathic care in the first few weeks."

Three months later, R.K. emailed me an image of herself standing in crampons on a glacier, with her weight on the side that used to hurt. The next month, her husband came in to shake my hand, looked into my eyes, and said with all his heart, "Thank you for giving my wife back to me."

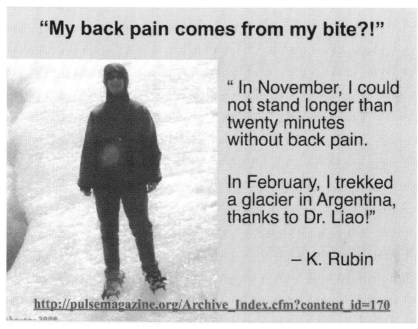

"My back pain comes from my bite?!"

" In November, I could not stand longer than twenty minutes without back pain.

In February, I trekked a glacier in Argentina, thanks to Dr. Liao!"

– K. Rubin

http://pulsemagazine.org/Archive_Index.cfm?content_id=170

Above: Post card from Antarctica glacier by RK.
Below: A basic oral appliance that helped RK's jaws, brain, and back.

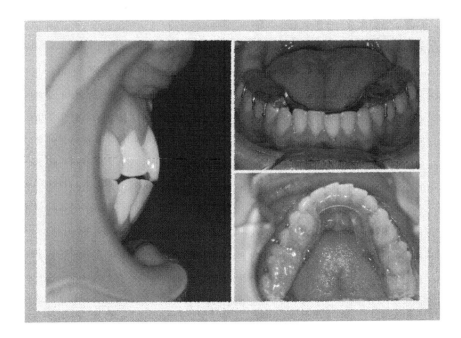

Holistic Mouth Means Alignment: The Law of Form and Function

An Impaired Mouth means misalignment and pain. Conversely, energy and vitality come naturally with alignment of the craniofacial-dental skeleton as follows:

A. Freedom from entrapped (retruded) position of maxilla and mandible relative to the cranium.

B. Sufficient width of both jaws to accommodate all teeth and the tongue between upper and lower arches.

C. Structural balance among the three key drivers of TMJ symptoms: maxilla position, front teeth angulation, and vertical dimension of occlusion, i.e. no deep overbite, nor open bite. [7]

D. The lower arch fitting into the upper as a foot fits into a shoe, with the upper arch as the shoe and the lower as the foot.

E. The head is mounted squarely over the Atlas, the top of

the neck. "When biomimetic oral appliance is used in combination with transdermal atlas repositioning, there appears to be a synergistic effect that significantly reduces LLD [leg length discrepancy] in adults." [8]

F. Balanced soft tissues connecting all the bones in the head i.e. no tongue tie, swollen tonsils, mouth breathing, nor swallowing with gurgling sound or grimaces around mouth, with oral-facial myofunctional therapy [9, 10]

G. Balanced soft tissues connecting head-jaws-spine-hips-legs-feet with cranio-sacral therapy, chiropractics, osteopathics, physical therapy, and acupuncture support. [11]

These are the structural requirements of Holistic Mouth, and the absence of TMJ dysfunction. Tandem teamwork is essential to produce sustainable outcome, as more cases ahead will show.

Holistic Mouth Nuggets:

- A is for Alignment in the ABCDES of Holistic Mouth. The cranio-facial-jaw bones have their own postural chain just like the spinal segments. Misalignment means TMJ pain and dysfunction, and vice versa.

- TMJ dysfunction can serve as another leading indicator of that familiar link from Impaired Mouth to deficient airway to poor sleep, and this is readily screened in routine dental checkup and cleaning visits.

- Bad back and bad bite can be connected, and a properly designed oral appliance can eliminate pain in both TMJ and beyond and related head-neck-back pain.

- Tandem treatment combining body work with oral appliances has been consistently effective to mitigate and even resolve chronic pain and fatigue. Being interested in your dental/oral health status is a sign of an integrative doctor/healthcare professional.

Chapter 14

Back Pain and Jaw Pain Go Poof — How Root Causes Are Found Treated in 3 case Studies

The best time to align the whole body is during dental makeover.

– Robert Walker, D.C., Founder of *Chirodontics*

Most doctors cannot fully appreciate the wisdom in Dr. Walker's quote above, let alone patients. That's because silo mentality by definition is limiting. Chiropractic adjustments are easily undone as long as malocclusion is not treated at the same time. That's because swallowing requires all teeth to be braced together, and swallowing saliva takes place about once a minute, or 1,440 times a day, not counting eating, drinking, and snacking/munching. That explains why chiropractics often do not hold.

Now let's see what can happen with tandem teamwork combining Holistic Mouth Solutions and chiropractic work as needed, instead.

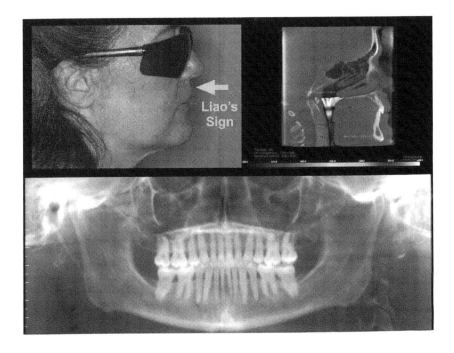

Still Hope for My Jaw Pain?

"Do you think there's still hope for my jaw pain at my age?" 45-year old Mrs. P. asked sheepishly one day at her son's bi-monthly oral appliance monitoring visit.

"So long as you have healthy teeth and no gum disease, age isn't a factor," I replied. "What are the three health symptoms you'd ask your Fairy Godmother to magically wave away? They can be medical, dental, or mental-emotional."

"Jaw pain with clicking when I open and close since I had braces as a 13-year old, for one. Those braces came after I had four adult teeth extracted. Number two? Back pain since I was 19," she continued. "And number three? Life-long anxiety."

Holistic Mouth evaluation revealed a limited jaw opening (35-40 mm instead of the optimal 48-51 mm) and trigger points in her jaw and neck muscles. Her MRI came back with a medical diagnosis of mild TMJ osteoarthritis on both sides and mild disk displacement of the left TMJ.

CT imaging showed that her airway was dangerously narrow 9 in the red-black zone), and cephalometric and model analyses both confirmed that extraction-retraction orthodontics had created a set of deficient jaws.

"Your deficient jaws are the cause of your narrow airway, which in turn creates oxygen deficiency and therefore your anxiety. Your Impaired Mouth has many ripple effects throughout your body. Cramps in your jaw-neck-back muscles is one of them."

"So, what can be done? I hope I don't need drugs or surgery."

"Let me figure out what's off, where, and by how much, and then I can give you a 'GPS' solution."

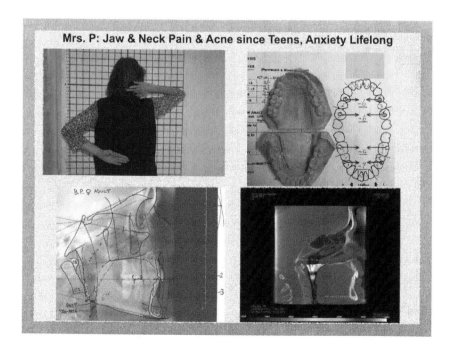

Mrs. P: Jaw & Neck Pain & Acne since Teens, Anxiety Lifelong

A week later, I reported to Mrs. P, "Your mouth volume decreased significantly after your extractions and their spaces were closed with braces," I continued. "Both of your jaws are retruded, so redeveloping your jaws FORWARD can make room in your mouth for your tongue. Both your pain and anxiety should get better when your jaws are redeveloped with oral appliances."

"Let's get started!"

Progress Report

Mrs. P. was highly compliant, which is vital to success. Treatment success is directly related to the wear time of the epigenetic oral appliance, as long as the diagnosis is correct and complete. Mrs. P. followed directions conscientiously and faithfully wore her appliances 14 to16 hours a day, including during sleep. She ate a healthy diet, walked for exercise, and kept her teeth and gums clean. How did she do?

- **One month:** "I am getting way more air and I can breathe through my nose better now. Flossing is getting easier — my teeth used to be so tight as to shred floss."

- **Two months:** "Clicking jaw sound is gone, and jaw pain is down 50%. I feel better with my appliances in my mouth."

- **Four months:** "Left ear throbbing is gone, when it used to be non-stop. It no longer comes on even when I am stressed. I have less daytime sleepiness, too."

- **Five months:** "All's good — no more TMJ pain, and no more back pain. I have more energy and mental clarity."

- **Six months:** "Back pain has not come back, and jaw pain is no longer the focal point my tension and stress."

- **Eight months:** "Dreaming way more and waking up energized. Tension in back of neck, left shoulder blade and right hand have come down with the combination treatment of chiropractics and oral appliances from 10 at their worst down to 1.5 with zero being no pain at all."

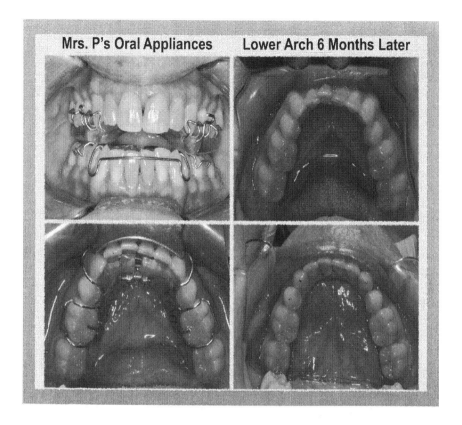

The lower arch should fit into the upper arch like a foot into a shoe. The tyranny of malocclusion goes poof when the lower front teeth are no longer crowded, i.e., the "toe box" is no longer deficient, and the upper arch is wide enough for the fully developed lower arch to fit in without retrusion.

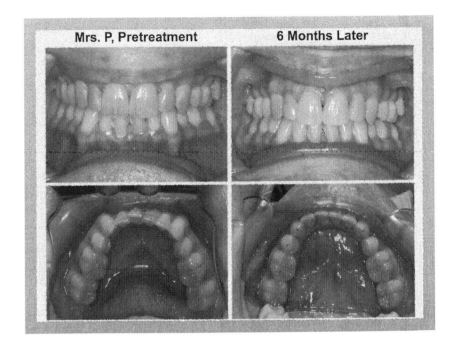

Mrs. P, Pretreatment | 6 Months Later

In a video recorded to help educate patients and doctors, Mrs. P. recounted her progress three months after starting treatment.

At the age of 19, I started to get TMJ pain off and on, so [there were] a lot of years of discomfort. And it slowly developed into neck and back pain and just an overall tension and lots of anxiety due to the stress of the pain and the tension in my jaw. My husband could hear the popping and clicking from across the room when I would eat.

And just from wearing both appliances for three months, I have no TMJ pain whatsoever. Now I have very little clicking and popping that was going on all the time…. I have no neck pain no back pain, and this is only after using both appliances for only three months. My anxiety is dramatically reduced. I can actually breathe through my nose. I can inhale and breathe.

I used to play in the band in high school, and when we marched, I really had a hard time breathing. I bet if I could do that now I would have no problem. So it's like I can actually do breathing exercises and get a lot more air in through my nose.

I have gone so many years in discomfort pain, and after only three months, it was just wiped away. It has been a fantastic experience.

A dentist trained as Holistic Mouth doctor can generate such results predictably.

Dentist's Son with TMJ Disorder

H.D. was referred to me by his mom, a dentist in another state. "My son is doing a postdoctoral study at the National Institutes of Health near you," she said. "He has this TMJ problem that I couldn't treat. Would you take a look at him for me?"

I did the same diagnostic workup for Impaired Mouth as described in earlier cases and concluded that oral appliance therapy could help H.D. After just one week with the appliance, he reported in a video testimonial:

> Before I got this DNA appliance, I was feeling lots of pain in my jaw, clicking popping, and discomfort and I couldn't eat without discomfort. After wearing this DNA appliance for one week, I feel a lot less pressure in my jaw area. It's done wonders for me.

Five years later, H.D. graduated from medical school. His Dr. Mom emailed me, "HD's been wearing the appliance you provided for him for the past 5 years! He says it has helped him and he's been wearing it at night."

To her credit, Dr. Mom has since shadowed me in my office and taken the necessary training. So, her patients have benefited from her son's TMJ problems, as well!

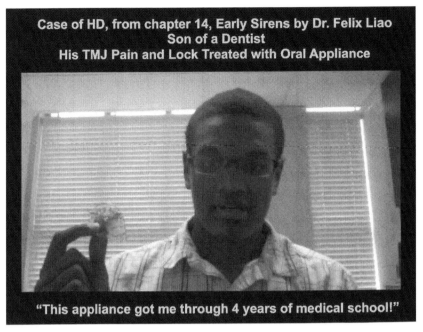

Video testimonials of Mrs. P, Daniel, and EJ are available online at www.HolisticMouthSolutions.com.

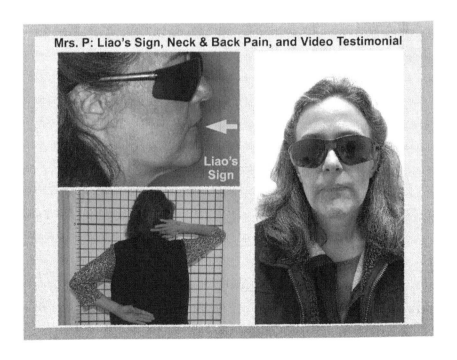

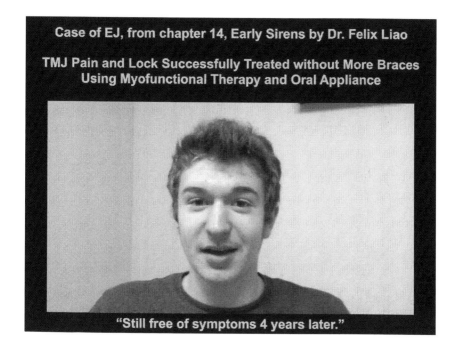

Case of EJ, from chapter 14, Early Sirens by Dr. Felix Liao

TMJ Pain and Lock Successfully Treated without More Braces Using Myofunctional Therapy and Oral Appliance

"Still free of symptoms 4 years later."

TMJ Problem Solved with Oral-facial Myofunctional Therapy: The Case of EJ

17-year-old E.J. was referred to me by his mom's chiropractor for a TMJ problem that came on 7 months after he had finished braces. "My jaw was locking up and popping when I opened my mouth and when I was chewing," he told me, "and that got very problematic." Mom was very concerned and upset.

Impaired Mouth diagnostics showed that braces had done a nice job of linking up E.J.'s teeth like boxcars on a railroad, but the rail beds needed work. In my report to his parents, I stated, "Jacob has well-aligned teeth from his orthodontic treatment – my compliments. In a nutshell, E.J.'s TMJ problem stems mainly from retruded jaws (opposite of protruded)."

Here's a most-overlooked principle: Align the jaws before you straighten the teeth. That means jaw orthopedics (bone-to-bone)

should come before orthodontics (teeth-to-teeth). The jaws need to be in alignment before the teeth can meet in harmony neurologically.

Simplicity is the rule here: Develop both jaws forward to free the TMJs from entrapment. Cephalometric analysis showed that E.J.'s lower jaw was bigger than his upper – the "foot" bigger than the "shoe."

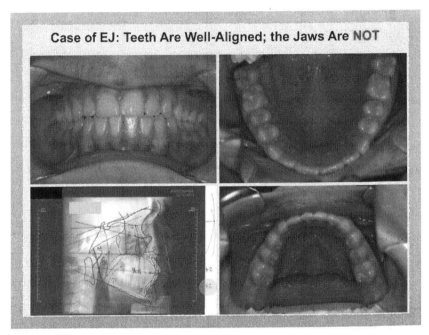

Orthodontics nicely done, but orthopedics were off,
which led to TMJ problem after EJ's braces

EJ's Holistic Mouth Solutions consisted of just 3 items: (A) simple oral appliance worn as much as possible, (B) sleep with an oral face mask, and (C) oral-facial myo-functional therapy, a set of exercises to reprogram the tongue, lips, cheeks, and throat muscles to adopt a more efficient pattern without side effects.

Three weeks after he began wearing his oral appliance, E.J. reported, "I felt great relief in my jaw after just two or three days, and it's been just great ever since." Mom added, "I'm just happy that we can avoid putting braces back on."

Four years later, E.J. was still free of his TMJ symptoms. "My jaw doesn't pop nearly as much and doesn't lock when I open my mouth straight up. I didn't used to be able to do this [opens mouth wide]."

Symptoms do not return when causes are identified and treated. TMJ problems are rooted in skeletal malocclusion, i.e., orthopedic misalignment of the jaws with the rest of head and neck.

Holistic Mouth Nuggets:

- Jaw clicking and TMJ-related pain is another useful early warning to health trouble(s) ahead. Root cause treatment is to free the mandible from its entrapment by redeveloping a deficient maxilla with Holistic Mouth Solutions™.

- Orthopedics comes before orthodontics: developing the jaws so the tongue fits comfortably between them should precede braces to straighten teeth. Braces with extraction of adult teeth contribute to chronic pain and fatigue, in my experience.

- Symptoms do not return when causes are identified and correctly treated through WholeHealth integration and tandem team treatment.

Chapter 15

Airway First – Find & Fix It Before Dental Implants or Reconstruction

These results... demonstrate the impossibility of dividing the patient up into neat little specialty areas to be treated without consideration of the resultant effects upon the total person, psyche and soma.

– Aelred C. Fonder, DDS, The Dental Physician [1]

Do you have failed root-canals in need of extraction or missing teeth in need of implants? Do you have a pattern of one dental trouble after another?

Since teeth are part of the Whole, dental failure means a decline in whole body health, which in turn is bad for the remaining teeth. Getting new teeth over dental implants can be a wonderful new start, but doing so without knowing *why* your natural teeth failed can get very expensive physically and financially.

Implants can be a god-send and very helpful – but may be risky in cases of jaw clenching and bruxing. Teeth grinding (sleep bruxism) carries a 3.4 times higher risk of implant failure. A 2016 Swedish study using international consensus sleep medicine metrics concludes that "bruxism was a statistically significantly risk factor to implant failure." [2]

Bone loss comes with each natural tooth loss and implant failure. Before starting implant work, be sure to ask, "Why did my natural tooth/teeth fail, and what's the cost of fixing failed implants and the resulting bone loss?" Beware if you are told that a night guard is the answer. As we saw earlier, defaulting to a night guard is a missed opportunity to assess the airway.

Remember ABC before XYZ — using the alphabets as analogy, Alignment-Breathing-Circulation comes before implants, which ranks in the neighborhood of XYZ, i.e., after the Impaired Mouth Syndrome is diagnosed and corrected.

Airway First

Airway rules because oxygen and sleep are not optional. That's why "Airway First" is THE guiding principle in my Holistic Mouth Solutions training seminars: Always check the patient's airway before starting treatment, be it dental, medical, nutritional, pharmaceutical, nutraceutical, or surgical.

As you have been learning, chronic oxygen deficiency from airway obstruction is a sure but much overlooked source of fatigue, pain, and sleep bruxing. This has implications for dental implants, as well.

Here is a sample of some of the science behind the bruxing-implants relationship:

- From a 1992 study: "Bone loss around implants after the first year... correlated well with the presence of overload..., teeth grinding or jaw clenching, and full mouth implants." [3]

- From a 2004 study: "Although dental implants have become a predictable aspect of tooth replacement... failures of up to 10% are still encountered." [4]

- From a 2016 study: "bruxism may be associated with an increased risk of dental implant failure." [5]

In addition, sleep bruxing comes with all the other adverse health impacts:

- Blood pressure surges 20 to 25 percent with sleep bruxing. [6]

- Sleep bruxing was present in 54 percent of mild OSA patients and 40 percent of moderate OSA patients, while another study reported that 25 percent of patients with sleep apnea have sleep bruxing. [7, 8]

- Teeth grinding stops when airway deficiency is restored. [9]

In my experience, neglecting Airway First before implant surgery can only lead to unhappy outcomes, as Ken's case shows next.

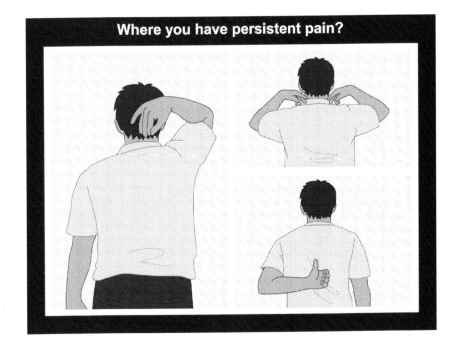

A Mouth-Body Disconnect: Ken's Story

"I can't sleep," said Ken, who was referred to me by a WholeHealth-minded acupuncturist, "and I have horrible neck pain that makes my eyes to glaze over. I've bought everything online that's promised to work, but nothing *has* worked. I am afraid of losing my job because I can't remember things."

Ken had socially desirable facial features and well-developed "beach muscles" from working out at his gym. But he could not get a date after meeting the single women he first connected with online. "They say my eyes scare them. I get this dazed look, like a deer caught in a car's headlight, when my pain would strike like an ice pick without warning out of nowhere."

What Ken's CSI (Chair Side Investigation) Revealed

"When did your pain begin?" I asked once it's clear what his presenting issues were. Long story short, a year before his pain started, Ken had all his upper teeth extracted. "I got sick and tired of them," he said, "because they were crowded, ugly, and nothing but trouble." He had his smile reconstructed with implants in one day at a cost of tens of thousands of dollars. Never was his airway assessed – nor his sinuses, neck, or, above all, the root cause of his upper teeth troubles.

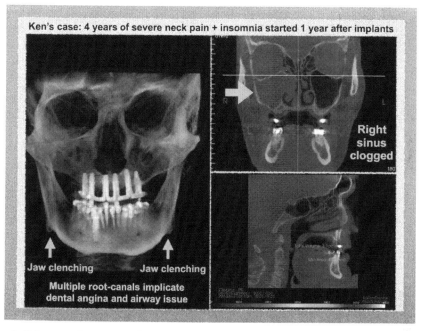

Left Image: 6 upper implants and 3 lower front root-canaled teeth are visible Upper right image: one sinus is completely clogged. Lower right image: Ken's airway is in the red-black zone, the extreme-trouble end of the color scale.

CT imaging showed that Ken had had seriously obstructed airway from a seriously deficient upper jaw, which offered only a size-one space for his size-six tongue. The replacement teeth Ken received duplicated his original malocclusion (bad bite) and thereby perpetuated his Impaired Mouth Syndrome and perhaps even aggravated his airway and sleep.

This was corroborated when a mandibular advance appliance improved sleep and mitigated his pain by holding his lower jaw forward during sleep. When Ken did not remember to wear his appliance, his pain and insomnia would come back in a flash.

The only non-surgical option left is a mandibular advancement appliance. Such appliances need to be worn for a lifetime, as it only compensates for a pinched airway overnight. Unfortunately, redeveloping the airway is not an option once teeth are pulled and implants placed. There are no stem cells left to turn on.

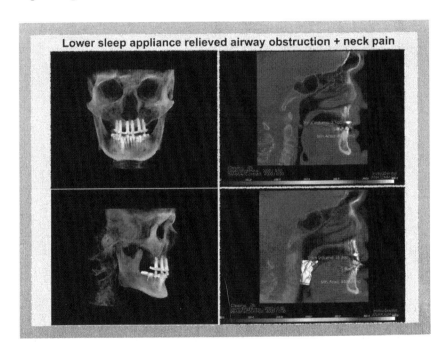

Lower sleep appliance relieved airway obstruction + neck pain

The Case of P.N.

"One of my patients broke her upper front bridge for the third time, and I have to fix it again," said a dentist enrolled in my Holistic Mouth Doctor training program. "Can you confirm my suspicion of an airway problem?"

"Yes, she likely has airway struggle during sleep, just by looking at the number of teeth lost, implants, and bridgework." I replied.

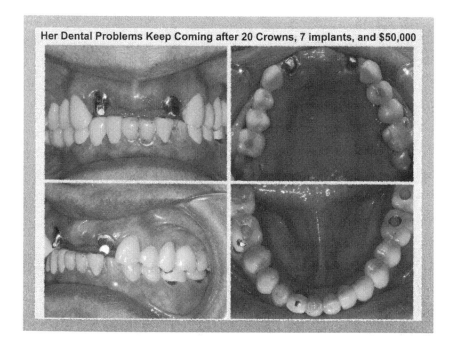

Her Dental Problems Keep Coming after 20 Crowns, 7 implants, and $50,000

Twenty of P.N.'s 28 adult teeth had been crowned. She had 7 implants and had lost 11 teeth total, including her two upper front teeth. These amount to big bucks to her dentist, but no corresponding benefits to her health.

Her oral hygiene was quite good, so plaque was not a likely cause of such tooth loss. But one look at her extremely narrow airway tells the WholeHealth story in her case.

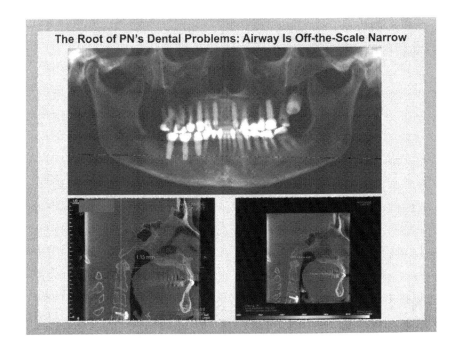

The Root of PN's Dental Problems: Airway Is Off-the-Scale Narrow

At intake, P.N. said that she experienced daytime sleepiness, fatigue, snoring, sleep apnea, teeth grinding, jaw clicking, and aches and pains in her neck and shoulders. "I'm on medication for high blood pressure," she added. Her hand was cold when we shook hands, and she admitted to unwanted weight gain despite her diet – both clues that medial evaluation for an underactive thyroid was in order.

"Your medical issues and dental problems may well be connected through the link of sleep-airway-mouth. I just wrote a book about this. Your health symptoms and dental troubles are likely reactions to sleeping with a six-foot tiger (your tongue) inside a three-foot cage (oral space between your jaws)."

"Really? That makes sense, but I wish my doctors had told me this years ago." P.N. shook her head in disappointment.

"Well, this is a new awareness just coming to light, thanks to advances in digital imaging, sleep medicine, and oral-systemic research. Making that sleep-airway-mouth connection can start helping you from having more dental troubles down the road, and possibly even a lessening of your medical symptoms."

"I can't wait to have no news as good news! How do I get started?"

"Start with reading my book *Six-Foot Tiger Three-Foot Cage* or bring your husband to my next monthly patient education talk. If you both agree, then we can start documenting your case with the necessary records such as CT scan, photos, and models to confirm the diagnosis of a narrow airway and deficient jaws. I can then figure out from your records what's off, where, and by how much, and recommend a customized Holistic Mouth Solutions to turn your mouth from a health lability into an asset."

"I look forward to reading your book, Dr. Liao."

"Thanks. But I am very sorry to tell you that yours is a very costly case. Your implants are very nicely done, but your airway does not support your teeth, nor your implants. Your current dental status does not support your total health. You have some infections from failing root-canaled still simmering, and you will likely need to replace most, if not all, of your old dental work."

"Why?" A look of concern comes of P.N.'s face.

"Airway should be fixed before implants. You don't move the furniture in until the foundation of the house is done and the room is finished. In your case, new furniture keeps getting delivered into your 'old Victorian' that has been falling apart structurally."

"Implants Comes After Airway"

This is worth repeating: ABC before XYZ — this is common sense not practiced in the rush to get new teeth in. Other thought leaders agree. "The teeth are the last piece of the Airway Centric paradigm. The airway is the first, then joint and muscle and, lastly, the occlusion", says TMJ expert Dr. Michael Gelb. [10]

In the case of P.N., having a wide-open airway can help not only her dental reconstruction but her heart, brain, and overall health, well-being, and bank account. These are the benefits of WholeHealth integration and Holistic Mouth solution. In the case of Ken, his memory affecting his work performance and job security, and his frustrating social life, both stem from his Impaired Mouth and Pinched airway undiagnosed.

When Impaired Mouth is detected and treated belatedly, both the savings account and whole body health pay a heavy price. When Impaired Mouth is detected and treated early enough, the whole body benefits.

If dental implant or reconstruction is coming up for you, remember to ask this question first: "What color is my airway, and can it support my WholeHealth?"

Holistic Mouth Nuggets

- Airway First means checking the airway before starting treatment, be it dental, medical, nutritional, pharmaceutical, nutraceutical, surgical, or implants. Neglecting the mouth-airway-sleep connections can be very expensive medically, dentally, financially, and socially.

- A narrow airway left undetected means a higher risk of failure is built into natural teeth and implant reconstruction.

- "One dental problem after another" leading to dental implants provides a series of early sirens to Impaired Mouth Syndrome's medical and dental complications. Fixing one failed tooth at a time can be far more costly in the end compared to diagnosing Impaired Mouth and treating it with Holistic Mouth Solutions™.

Chapter 16

Impaired Brain from Impaired Mouth: Proactive Response to Your Early Sirens

It's fair to say that the person you are when you're awake is partly a function of what your brain does when you're asleep.

– Ken Paller, PhD [1]

What's the most important supplement for the brain? It's oxygen, not fish oil, in my experience. More than any other part of your body, your brain needs oxygen to stay well and thrive. We can go for days without food and water but only minutes without oxygen. That is how an Impaired Mouth and its pinched airway contribute to brain degeneration and mental health issues.

That is also why a Holistic Mouth Checkup on your jaws and airway is important to your brain's well-being. Nutritional therapy and functional medicine for brain health starts with airway and sleep, which means Airway First, just like dental implants.

Just as treating toothache in time as dental angina can rescue a toothache from root-canal treatment (chapter 11), early recognition of Impaired Mouth Syndrome holds the promise to heading off premature brain degeneration.

Trained Holistic Mouth Doctors: First-Line Diagnosticians

Loss of eye sight, teeth, and memory rank among patients' greatest fears, and you now know that Impaired Mouth contributes to all three through diabetes, teeth grinding, and sleep apnea.

Dentists trained as doctors of Holistic Mouth can be first-line diagnosticians to connect the dots, screen for early clues of more serious health troubles ahead, educate patients, refer appropriately, or institute proactive solutions. Checkup visits every 6 months makes the dental office an ideal place for screening, provided the attending doctor has left the conventional dentistry silo and made the paradigm shift from teeth to mouth.

Alzheimer's disease is on the mind of many of my patients caring for their afflicted and aging parents. It takes 15-20 years for memory loss to show up, but it may be too late by then to reverse the damage. The more sensible step is to wake up to the early sirens coming from your Impaired Mouth at every 6-month dental checkup visit that doubles as a Holistic Mouth screening. Let's now connect impaired brain with the established link of impaired mouth-airway-sleep.

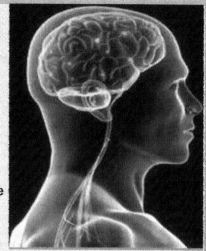

Impaired mouth can contribute to these symptoms:

- Teeth grinding
- Bladder urgency
- Morning headaches
- Daytime sleepiness
- Aches and pains, fatigue
- Pot belly, double chin
- Brain fog, poor memory
- Depression, anxiety
- High blood pressure

Mouth doctors can be first-line diagnosticians.

The High Cost of Alzheimer's Disease

As of 2013, the disease ranked sixth among America's leading causes of death. [2] The cost of caring for this "long good-bye" deserves everyone's attention, especially those who do not sleep well and those with family members with sleep apnea signs and symptoms but without treatment.

According to the Alzheimer's Association, "Dementia costs more to American society than heart disease and cancer – and is now the most expensive disease in the United States – according to an NIH-funded study recently published in the *New England Journal of Medicine.* The study found that with the aging of the baby boomers, the costs of dementia are expected to skyrocket.[3]. This has big implications for Medicare and state budgets and your retirement alike.

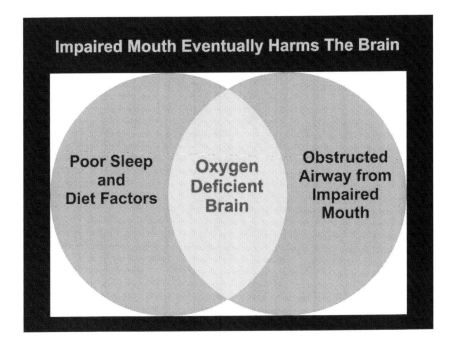

Oxygen Deficiency Means Chronic Stress to the Brain

Living with an Impaired Mouth and sleeping with a pinched airway amounts to burning the proverbial candle from both ends. One end is the lack of rest and regeneration from poor sleep, and the other is brain damage from oxygen deprivation.

Waking up tired does not bode well for the day, nor down the road for the part of the brain that deals with memory, the *hippocampus*. As one study in *BMC Neuroscience* explains, "The hippocampus is essential for declarative memory synthesis and is a core pathological substrate for Alzheimer's disease (AD), the most common aging-related dementing disease. Acute increases in plasma [blood] cortisol are associated with transient hippocampal inhibition and retrograde amnesia, while chronic cortisol elevation is associated with hippocampal atrophy." [4]

Translation: Stress harms memory. This explains the experience of "I can't think just now!" when an overwhelming stressor suddenly strikes. But how about long-term stress on brain memory, as in sleeping with airway obstructed inside an Impaired Mouth year after year?

Cortisol level is an indicator chronic stress. A 2009 study from Taiwan reported that "elevated levels of plasma cortisol predicted a worse general cognitive performance. Higher plasma cortisol levels also correlated with rapid declines in MMSE [mini-mental state evaluation] scores after 2 years. The relationship between high cortisol levels and hippocampal atrophy might adversely affect AD patients disproportionately, either in anatomical or cognitive function." [5]

Airway obstruction during sleep is a form of chronic stress impacting every part of the body, especially the brain. Here is some eye-popping data: "Aging induced a 12% decrease in hippocampus activity, increased to 30% by acute and 40% by chronic elevations in cortisol... suggesting a chronic elevation in cortisol may be more detrimental in this system rather than an acute elevation," according to a 2009 study from UK's Newcastle University. [6]

Translation: The risk for Alzheimer's disease from chronic stress is 3.5 times greater than from aging alone. Given the bankruptcy potential of Alzheimer's on personal, state, and national levels, doesn't it make sense to attend to the early sirens coming from the mouth?

Impaired Mouth > Sleep Apnea > Impaired Brain

An Impaired Mouth eventually harms your teeth, heart, and brain, and it costs you every step along health's downhill slide. Oral contributions to brain degeneration can include gum disease, oral infections, and choked airway.

Both Alzheimer's and periodontal infections are impacted by the oxygen deprivation. Pinched airway means less oxygen, which in turn favors the bad gram-negative pathogens that turns on gum inflammation. Gum disease is the major cause of tooth loss in adults. A small sample of the science of oral-systemic links include:

- Elderly women with sleep apnea are twice as likely to develop Alzheimer's disease or other forms of dementia within five years, compared with women without, according to a University of California study. [7, 8]

- Oxygen deprivation contributes to cognitive impairment. According to a study in BMC Neuroscience, "Elevated oxygen desaturation index (more than 15 events/hour) and high percentage of sleep time (over 7%) in apnea or hypopnea (both measures of disordered breathing) were associated with risk of developing mild cognitive impairment or dementia." [9]

- "Sustained, long-term CPAP [continuous positive airway pressure] treatment for patients with Alzheimer's and OSA may result in lasting improvements in sleep and mood as well as a slowing of cognitive deterioration," concludes a 2009 study on CPAP treatment. [10]

- A study in the Journal of the American Geriatrics Society found that "OSA treatment seems to improve some cognitive functioning. Clinicians who care for Alzheimer's disease patients should consider implementing CPAP treatment when OSA is present." [11]

- A Korean study found "a significant association between OSA and periodontal disease" in subjects who were 55 years of age or older. "The results showed that 17.5 percent of the participants had periodontitis…and 60.0 percent who were diagnosed with periodontitis had OSA." [12]

- A 2012 study from New York University College of Dentistry concluded "Periodontal inflammation may affect cognition."[13]

- Inflammation around the gum line or bleeding when brushing and flossing does not bode well for your brain either. As a 2016 study in PLoS Medicine put it, "Our data showed that periodontitis is associated with an increase in cognitive decline in Alzheimer's Disease, independent to baseline cognitive state, which may be mediated through effects on systemic inflammation." [14]

All of these findings make Holistic Mouth Checkup in a dental office every 6 month a most efficient place to screen for Alzheimer's risk and to "recalculate" for an alternate route to its hazards ahead.

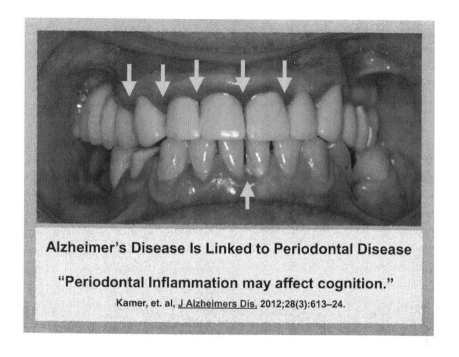

Alzheimer's Disease Is Linked to Periodontal Disease

"Periodontal Inflammation may affect cognition."

Kamer, et. al, J Alzheimers Dis. 2012;28(3):613–24.

"Anxious and Depressed and I Don't Know Why": B.D.'s Story

B.D. was in her early sixties when she came to see me. Her presenting complaints started with (a) waking tired every day of the week "since forever", and (b) weakening memory. "I have to write everything down now," she said, "or I will forget."

Medically, she had stomach and mood problems. "I get really anxious and depressed, and I don't know why." She also had pain in her back, shoulders, and neck.

Dentally, she could not chew well anymore because she had lost so many teeth. B.D.'s panoramic x-ray showed five root-canals remaining, six molars lost (not counting wisdom teeth), and at least two more teeth with so much bone loss to gum disease that soon she'd be without any teeth on her upper right side.

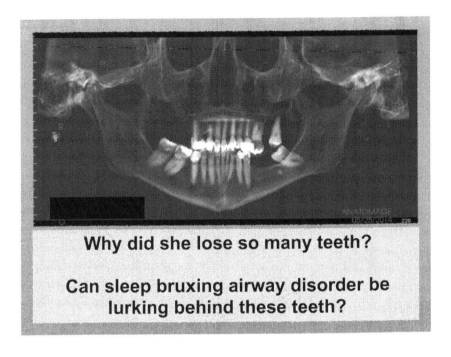

Why did she lose so many teeth?

Can sleep bruxing airway disorder be lurking behind these teeth?

The WholeHealth mind asks: can all those symptoms be connected? Yes – from living with a six-foot tiger in a three-foot cage that had never been diagnosed. Her doctors and dentists cannot be blamed because they had not been trained to connect the medical-dental dots via the airway.

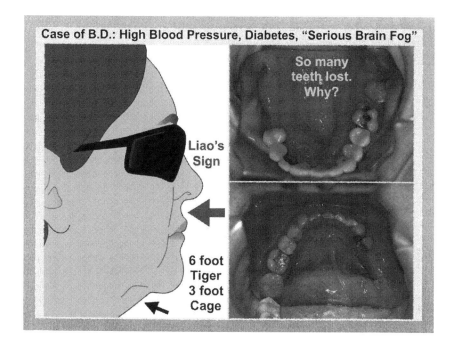

Case of B.D.: High Blood Pressure, Diabetes, "Serious Brain Fog"

B.D.'s teeth were squeaky-clean, her tooth loss is not likely due to poor oral hygiene. So, what could explain it? B.D. had a narrow Zone 3 on her CT scan. Her oral airway volume was about one-quarter of low normal. That explained her constant anxiety — she could never get enough air through her very pinched airway.

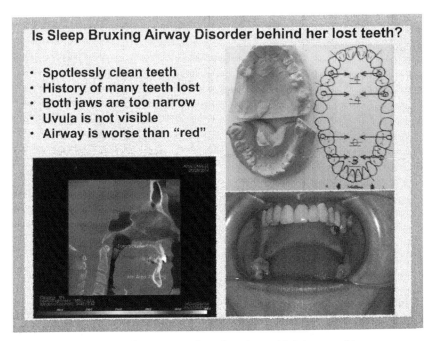

Teeth grinding is now sleep bruxing, which is rooted in clogged airway inside an Impaired Mouth

Impaired Mouth Led to Medical-Dental-Mental Symptoms

B.D.'s impaired mouth just could not support sleep and total health. She had Liao's sign, suggesting retruded maxilla. Her airway was choked because her jaws were undeveloped and narrow. I suspected that sleep bruxing was the likely cause of her continuing tooth loss despite excellent home care and good dental work.

B.D.'s fatigue and memory symptoms came in major part from having lived with oxygen deficiency 24/7 for over fifty years. During that time, she had gone to dentists regularly and kept her teeth and gums very clean, yet she kept losing one tooth after another. To be fair, sleep medicine is much more advanced now, and dentists back in the old days did not have any dots to connect, much less solutions to offer.

From the WholeHealth perspective, B.D. has four mercury-containing amalgam fillings which appear graying-black suggesting corrosion over a long time. Airway comes first, but teeth with infections and toxic fillings also cause the mouth to block whole body health. Here's a brief glimpse at this vastly overlooked source of perplexing symptoms resistant to treatment before we return to sleep-airway-mouth connection to the brain.

A 2010 study published in Journal of Alzheimers Disease (AD) did a systematic review of 1,041 references from forty studies concluded:

- "Mercury is one of the most toxic substances known to humans;

- 32 studies out of 40 testing memory in individuals exposed to inorganic mercury, found significant memory deficits;

- In vitro models showed that inorganic mercury reproduces all pathological changes seen in AD;

- Inorganic mercury may play a role as a co-factor in the development of AD." [15]

"Higher mercury concentrations were found in brain regions and blood of some patients with Alzheimer's disease (AD)... Mercury levels in brain tissues are 2 - 10 fold higher in individuals with dental amalgam.", reports a 2007 study from Germany. "Main human sources for mercury are fish consumption (Methyl-Hg) and dental amalgam (Hg vapor). Regular fish consumption reduces the risk of development of AD." [16]

Mercury amalgam's toxic effect is not limited to the brain. A small sample of studies linking heart disease to toxic teeth include:

- "Mercury has a high affinity for sulfhydryl groups... [thereby] inactivating numerous enzyme reactions... with subsequent decreased oxidant defense and increased oxidative stress... Mercury toxicity should be evaluated in any patient with hypertension, coronary heart disease, cerebral vascular disease, cerebrovascular accident, or other vascular disease", reports a 2011 study from Vanderbilt Medical School. [17]

- "A large increase of over 10,000 times (of mercury and antimony) of TE [trace element] concentration has been observed in myocardial but not in muscular samples in all pts with idiopathic dilated cardiomyopathy." [18].

- "The findings presented here suggest that mercury poisoning from dental amalgam may play a role in the etiology of cardiovascular disorders. Comparisons between subjects with and without amalgam showed amalgam-bearing subjects had significantly higher blood pressure, lower heart rate... [and] a greater incidence of chest pains, tachycardia, anemia, fatigue, tiring easily, and being tired in the morning. The data suggest that inorganic mercury poisoning from dental amalgam does affect the cardiovascular system." [19]

"I know you can find numerous dentists and physicians that will say amalgams are not a risk factor for AD---see if you can find one that will debate me publicly after allowing me to present a short scientific talk on the subject. I feel like I have been in an 8 year argument with a town drunk on this issue", wrote Dr. Boyd Haley, Professor and chair Department of Chemistry at University of Kentucky. "I strongly believe that having a dental amalgam in one's mouth for scores of years increases the risk for AD.... because I read the literature and do research in this area... the bottom line is that amalgams make both water and saliva toxic by increasing mercury levels... I hope you know that AD is not a directly inherited disease and that some form of 'toxic or infective insult' is needed to cause the onset of the disease." [20] A rich reference on mercury-amalgam toxicity is available from Dr. Tom McGuire. [21]

A strong caution: mercury is a potent environmental and neurological toxin. And If you have mercury amalgam in your teeth and you have medical concerns over your brain health, be sure to have it removed in a MERCURY-SAFE manner by choosing only dentists who have had proper training to protect you and themselves from www.IABDM.org, www.IAOMT.org, or International Association of Mercury Safe Dentists (IAMSD). The American Dental

Association's protocol is limited in scope in comparison with the above, but it supports mercury-safe practice in principle. [22]

Dentists not trained in mercury-safe practices suffer from brain and other neurological damage more than their patients:

- Amalgam consists of approx. 50 % of elementary mercury which is constantly being vaporized and absorbed by the organism." [23]

- "Chronic inhalation of low-level Hg0 [mercury vapor from amalgam fillings at mouth temperature] can inhibit polymerization of brain tubulin essential for formation of microtubules." [24]

Dentists are exposed to mercury by virtue of going through dental school and looking into the mouths of patients with amalgam fillings. In light of such evidence, dentists who are themselves victims of mercury toxicity may want to recuse themselves from arguing that "mercury from amalgams is not a problem" until they are declared mercury-free by a qualified medical doctor.

Going forward, however, keeping B.D.'s teeth would not be hard, but rebuilding would be very costly. She did not come back after I showed her my findings and analysis. The cost of dental reconstruction alone in such cases can be a non-starter. This is an issue that America's health insurance system must address as Baby Boomers continue aging.

What other clues are there on the way to cognitive decline and other brain impairments?

"Tired and Depressed": H.N.'s Story

Another recurrent theme among new patients who come to see me is their feeling perpetually "tired and depressed". Sleep issues are commonly the cause. As the Harvard Sleep Health Center notes, "Chronic sleep issues have been correlated with depression, anxiety, and mental distress." [25]

Sleep and Mood Disorders

http://healthysleep.med.harvard.edu/need-sleep/whats-in-it-for-you/mood

- 1/3 - 1/2 of pts with chronic sleep problems have mood disorders

- Insomnia = 20X risk for anxiety

- Insomnia = 10X risk for depression

- Difficulty sleeping is sometimes the first symptom of depression

- "People who have problems with sleep are at increased risk for developing emotional disorders, depression, and anxiety."

Dr. Lawrence Epstein, Medical Director of Harvard Sleep Health Centers

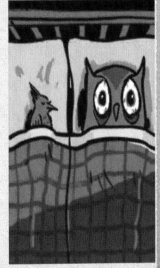

Illustration by Nishant Choksi

According the Centers for Disease Control and Prevention, "Depression is characterized by depressed or sad mood, diminished interest in activities which used to be pleasurable, weight gain or loss, psychomotor agitation or retardation, fatigue, inappropriate guilt, difficulties concentrating, as well as recurrent thoughts of death." [26]

But depression is more than just having a "bad day." Diagnostic criteria established by the American Psychiatric Association dictate that five or more of the above symptoms must be present for a continuous period of at least two weeks." [27]

Moreover, "Depression appears to be associated with poor sleep throughout the lifespan." [28, 29] Yet antidepressant medications rank among the most prescribed drugs today. Only you can answer this question: "Would I choose to treat the cause, or compensate for the symptoms?"

H.N. was referred by her WholeHealth-minded psychiatrist who saw that sleep and airway could be important factors in her depression. At age 27, H.N. had been depressed for over twenty years. On her initial visit, her face showed all the signs of impaired mouth: double chin, thick neck, and obesity in the head, neck, trunk and thighs. She had a swollen tongue suggestive of thyroid dysfunction. Her uvula was not visible, and her maxilla was V-shaped. Liao's Sign was apparent, implicating retruded jaws and a pinched airway. Her front teeth showed matching wear facets, confirming a likely sleep bruxing airway disorder.

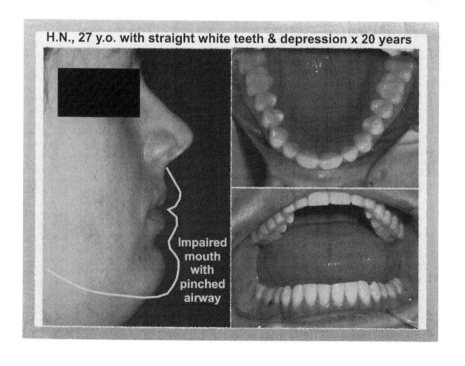

H.N., 27 y.o. with straight white teeth & depression x 20 years

Impaired mouth with pinched airway

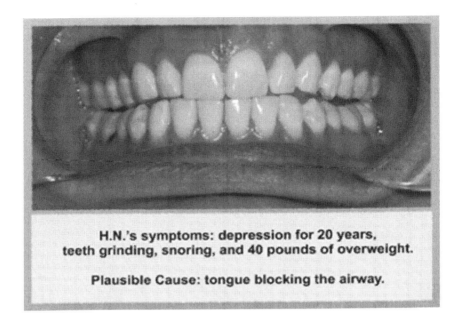

H.N.'s symptoms: depression for 20 years, teeth grinding, snoring, and 40 pounds of overweight.

Plausible Cause: tongue blocking the airway.

H.N. had been on CPAP based on a prior sleep test, and she elected to start oral appliance therapy. At her one week follow-up visit, she reported a significant improvement in her quality of life already.

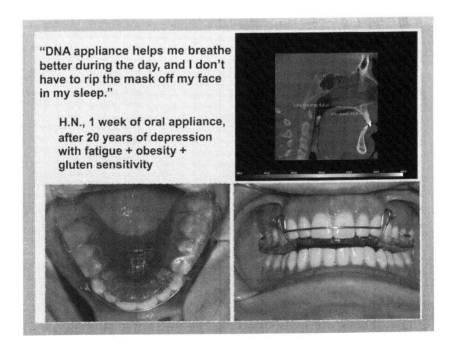

"DNA appliance helps me breathe better during the day, and I don't have to rip the mask off my face in my sleep."

H.N., 1 week of oral appliance, after 20 years of depression with fatigue + obesity + gluten sensitivity

Compared to B.D., H.N. was more fortunate to have her impaired mouth recognized and her airway treated early on so that she could avoid B.D.'s medical and dental problems later.

Oral Herpes Infections: Another Clue Warning of Alzheimer's Risk

Catching a cold means the immune system is down. So is a "cold sore", which is caused by Herpes Simplex virus (HSV). HSV normally resides dormant our nervous system. Oral cold sores pop up on the lips, the gums, cheeks, tongue, or throat, when the stress of unhealthy lifestyle and/or airway obstruction night after night takes its toll.

Interestingly, studies have shown the HSV1 strain has been linked to increased risk for Alzheimer's disease:

- A 2008 British study reported: "there is strong evidence that the virus is indeed a major factor in AD [Alzheimer's disease]" acting "in combination with a genetic factor." [30]

- Another 2008 study from France concluded, "HSV chronic infection may therefore be contributive to the progressive brain damage characteristic of AD. Controlled for age, gender, educational level and Apolipoprotein E4 (APOE4) status, IgM-positive subjects [infected with HSV] showed a significant higher risk of developing AD, with a hazard ratio of 2.55." [31]

Translation: if 2 siblings both with the Alzheimer gene, the one with oral herpes sores from HSV1 will have more than 2.5 times the risk for developing the disease.

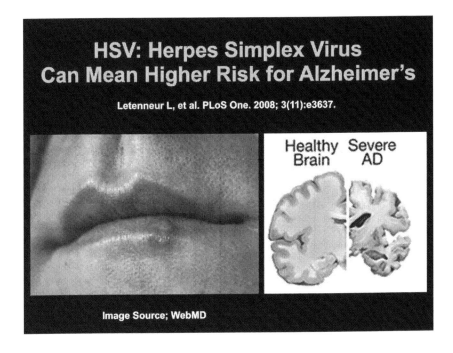

Sleep is a natural solution to reboot the immune army against the invading or resident virus — provided the airway is not obstructed. That's why it's important to know if you are suffering from Impaired Mouth Syndrome.

Help Your Brain the WholeHealth Way

Sleepy healthy is more important than eating healthy in this increasingly toxic world, in my view. A WholeHealth approach means addressing *all* facets of lifestyle that affect health for better or worse. For example, exercise can cut Alzheimer's risk by half. [32]

For some excellent tips on taking a proactive, preventive approach to Alzheimer's, see Dr. David Perlmutter's "Drug Free Approach Cuts Alzheimer's Risk in Half" at GreenMedInfo.com. [33]

Ultimately, supplying the brain with all the oxygen it needs during sleep is a sensible and promising way to keep the brain neurons from turning blue and purple. In severe sleep apnea cases, this can be done with CPAP. In mild to moderate cases, oral appliance therapy can get the job done, and the earlier the better.

The pattern of impaired mouth, gum inflammation, tooth loss, and pinched airway is emerging to be a contributor to Alzheimer's disease. See a Holistic Mouth doctor early to avoid it.

Holistic Mouth Nuggets

- Dementia, memory loss, depression, and other brain and mental health issues are associated with poor sleep and sleep disordered breathing. Waking up tired does not bode well for today, nor brain health down the road. Don't wait until memory loss to get your Holistic Mouth checkup.

- Airway obstruction during sleep can explain why some people never recover once they fall ill. Deep sleep can resolve or mitigate many symptoms naturally, but it depends on a wide-open airway.

- The risk for Alzheimer's disease from chronic stress is 3.5 times greater than from aging alone. Undiagnosed and untreated Impaired Mouth Syndrome may be a major source of chronic stress from sleeping with choked airway.

Chapter 17

Chair Side Investigations:
Finding the Missing Link to
Restart and Renew Your Health

A Holistic Mouth approach is far beyond 'drill, fill, and bill' dentistry as we doctors and patients know it. Good oral hygiene is essential, but no amount of brushing and flossing will fix the symptoms of Impaired Mouth Syndrome.

– John Trowbridge, MD,
Author of *The Yeast Syndrome, and Sick and Tired?*

All too often, the mouth is left out in medical-dental treatment plans and hospital care. This can make the quest for health and wellness very expensive, as the patients in these pages have taught us. Patchwork care fixes symptoms but leaves the cause untouched so new trouble and sprout again later.

WholeHealth is the necessary integration of mind-body-mouth to make all the parts and systems work as a seamless whole. Let's see how this line of thinking can trace the clues back to watershed source of persistent illness resistant to otherwise effective treatment.

Chair Side Investigation (CSI): Clues + Knowledge

CSI begins with the WholeHealth view of the patient. In the care of health, every CSI starts with this opening question: "Is this body getting what it needs to get well or stay well? If not, what's in the way?"

Through this kind of Chair Side Investigation, we connect the dots and trace symptoms back to their root causes. Think of Sherlock Holmes astutely picking up clues overlooked by others at the crime scene. Finding the culprit requires constructing a plausible working hypothesis based on the clues, logic, and having an impressive database of knowledge.

The same goes with solving Impaired Mouth Syndrome. The dentist-turned Holistic Mouth doctor needs to be able to detect clues and put the puzzle pieces back together with WholeHealth knowledge covering mind-body-mouth-lifestyle and more. The same goes for physicians and other non-dental health professionals.

Consider how a newborn grows: repeated cycles of sleeping and feeding until it gains enough strength to hold up their head and use their hands. Sleep, airway, nutrition, rest would be the answers to that opening question. Sometimes, asking one critical question can be the difference-maker, as you'll see in the case of Jenna.

OneLook YouKnow™: Big Clue to Start CSI

"Nothing has really helped, and I'm getting worse by the day." Jenna, age 43 and a nursing school instructor, came to see me with a neck collar on and cane in hand. Her husband had brought her to me for a Holistic Mouth consultation.

"A year ago, I suffered a traumatic brain injury from overhead filming equipment." During that time, she saw over twenty-five doctors. Still, her condition deteriorated. At times, she needed a wheelchair to get around.

One look at her and I knew she had been suffering from undiagnosed Impaired Mouth Syndrome: She had what I call Liao's Sign – a flat or curled upper lip in profile, which I have found to be a regular facial feature in patients with an Impaired Mouth and a pinched airway inside.

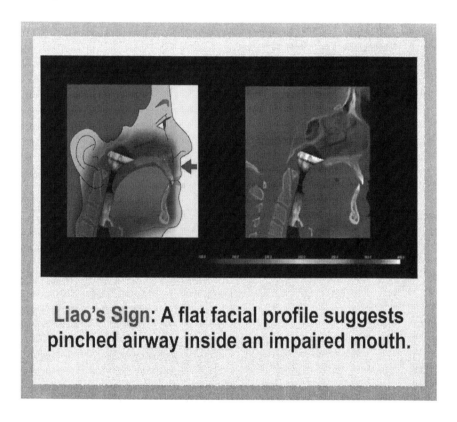

Liao's Sign: A flat facial profile suggests pinched airway inside an impaired mouth.

As I describe it in *Six-foot Tiger, Three-foot Cage*:

- Liao's Sign is a "rule of thumb" facial indicator of a retruded upper jaw that belies an impaired mouth. Retrusion is the opposite of protrusion. A retruded maxilla frequently results in a narrower airway behind the soft palate.

- A positive Liao's sign implicates a deficient airway until proven otherwise. Yet the absence of Liao's sign does not mean all is well. A non-retruded maxilla can still be too narrow and lead to a "three-foot cage" from having teeth taken out for braces and the resulting spaces closed with braces, and other causes.

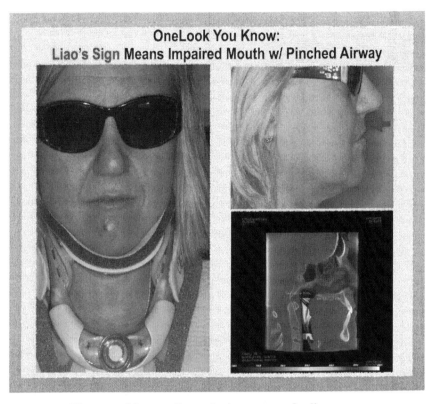

The case of Jenna: Airway in the green and yellow range is still too deficient to support her health.

"How's your thyroid status?" I asked Jenna. "Your hand was ice cold when we shook hands."

"I'm on medical thyroid supplement now, but it took three years to normalize me. I've had lifelong constipation, and gluten and dairy sensitivities."

"They're often related, and it seems to me your thyroid status still can use some upgrade. Please check with your doctor." I said before asking, "What's happened to you since your traumatic brain injury?"

"My mind is less clear. My recall is less. I need a cane to keep my balance when I stand. My sleep quality has gone drastically downhill. I wake up four or five times a night."

"Any significant dental problems in your history?"

"I've had a night guard for teeth grinding and TMJ problem since as long as I can remember."

"That's another footprint at our 'crime scene' that can lead us toward the culprit. Any aches and pains?"

"Both hips, shoulders and neck. I needed monthly massages."

"How's your digestion?"

"I'm a vegetarian. I have zero ability to digest protein, and I have a severely limited food list."

In WholeHealth, all these clues are interconnected. In patchwork care, there's one doctor for every condition, but rarely is the patient a functional Whole.

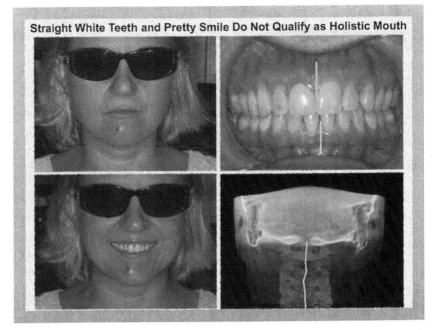

Straight White Teeth and Pretty Smile Do Not Qualify as Holistic Mouth

Misalignment of dental midlines means neck misalignment, uneven blood supply to the brain, and aches and pains in head-jaws-neck-shoulders and beyond.

The Key to Recovery: How's Your Sleep?

"The twenty-five top notch doctors you have consulted can't all be wrong. Something is stopping them from being totally right," I said to Jenna's most supportive husband.

"We're hoping you can tell us." He said.

"How was your sleep before your accident?" I asked Jenna.

"It was never good." She shrugged and smiled at the same time.

"That may be the key to your recovery. The body knows how to fix itself 95% of the time when it can get into deep sleep. That's when the full healing power of God or Nature is downloaded into your body. So, let's see if we can help you into deeper sleep by opening up your airway."

"Is that done with your oral appliances?"

"Yes. Oral appliances have the potential of helping with your sleep *and* pain because your dental midlines are off."

Jenna started oral appliance therapy to correct her deficient and misaligned jaws as part of her Holistic Mouth Solutions. Here's Jenna's progress:

> **Week 1:** "Sleep more and clarity of thoughts improved, and both eyes are tracking better."
>
> **Month 1:** "TMJ pain is down, neck pain is down by 50%, and walking is improved. No longer feel the need to wear neck brace."
>
> **Month 3:** "Sleeping 12 hours a day and waking feeling refreshed."
>
> **Month 4:** "Giant cognitive difference in the last 2 months." Her husband C.J. added that she was no longer snoring.
>
> **Month 5:** "Incredible changes since Dr. Liao's work," wrote C.J. "Now she can walk much better, and can read now, and she has started to take back the household tasks, all of which she could not do after the accident."

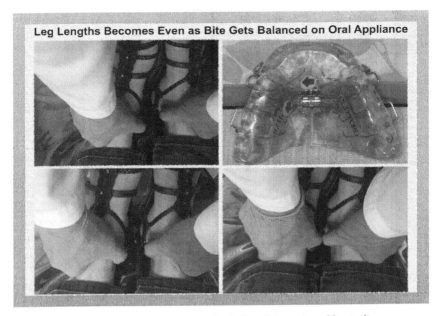

Leg Lengths Becomes Even as Bite Gets Balanced on Oral Appliance

The doctor's thumb pads over the balls of Jenna's ankles indicate her leg length. Counter-clockwise from top left: leg length becomes even after bite on oral appliance is balanced.

This Holistic Mouth CSI tells us exactly why her prior treatments had failed and revealed the root cause of her suffering: an undiagnosed Impaired Mouth structure. It starts with observing Liao's sign, moves to asking, "How's your sleep?" then gets confirmation on the pinched airway and jaw-neck alignment.

Her CSI also guided Jenna's Holistic Mouth Solutions™: cranio-sacral therapy, acupuncture, a single maxillary (upper) oral appliance for 16 hours a day, and an oral face mask during sleep. She has found wearing it full-time (except to eat) makes her feel better.

Cranio-Sacral Therapy

While the cranium is the bony enclosure that houses the brain, the sacrum is a triangular shape bone between the hip bones that form the pelvis which houses your lower digestive tract and your urinary and reproductive organs. The cranio-sacral system covers us literally from head to tail bone.

Cranio-sacral therapy originates in the osteopathic tradition of gently easing stuck or displaced skull bones into alignment. It began with Dr. William Sutherland, who was inspired by the beveled sutures joining the parietal and the temporal bones of the cranium. He thought they are meant for breathing motions "like the gills of a fish."

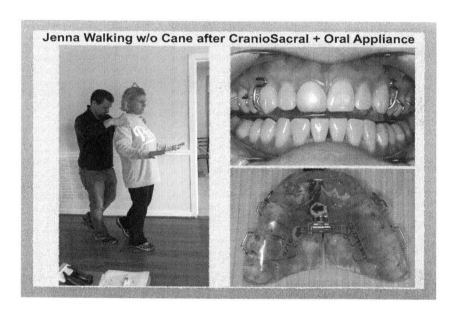

Dr. Sutherland called that subtle breathing motion *primary respiration*, which is like the pulse of the central nervous system. He found that sick people had impaired cranial respiration and that they could be made well by very gently manipulating the displaced/stuck cranial bone(s) back into place, and thereby restore their primary respiration.

Osteopathic physician Dr. John Upledger took Dr. Sutherland's cranial osteopathy and developed it into cranial-sacral therapy in the 1970s. *Craniosacral rhythm* become the new term for primary respiration.

Cranio-sacral therapy (CST) is a very light-touch treatment and highly relaxing. In my experience, it feels like having your entire body's hardwiring reset to "human." But it's not just a touchy-feely treatment. Cranial-sacral rhythm is as basic to health as sleep and airway.

The cranium is not a hard coconut shell as many still think today. Brain cells actually "breathe" in a subtle but palpable rhythmic manner, and the brain case comes with cranial sutures to accommodate this cranial-sacral rhythm. It feels like a gentler baby version of inhale-exhale of chest breathing. With training, you can feel it on the ankles, pelvis, collar bone, or anywhere in the body. You'd be in awe once you learn to sense this subtle but vital expression of life and intelligence.

Good form is a prerequisite for good function and good health. Symptoms and disorders show up the cranial bone's joints (sutures) are slipped or stuck. Cranio-sacral therapy provides the right cranial structural form for the central nervous system to work effectively.

From Cranial Form to Neurological Functions

For patients with palatal asymmetry, uneven eyes, ears, TMJ disorder, persistent pain, chronic fatigue, and lingering illness, CST can be invaluable in combination with oral appliance therapy as part of the WholeHealth-oriented Holistic Mouth Solution, as Jenna's case shows.

Conditions which CST can help include post-concussion symptoms, migraines and headaches, chronic neck and back pain, stress- and tension-related disorders, TMJ syndrome, scoliosis, ADD/ADHD, chronic fatigue, and more. [2]

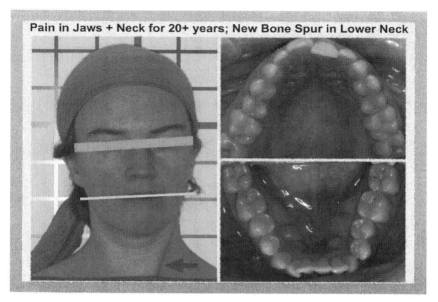

Above: head-jaw misalignment means neck pain and postural distortion. Note the right-left asymmetry of her upper and lower dental arches.

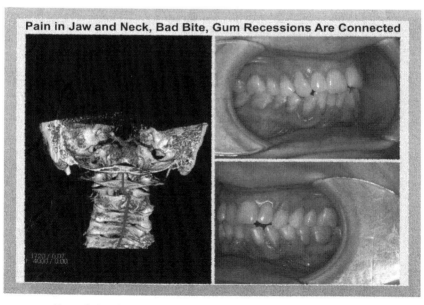

Above left: The neck frequently pays the price of pain when the jaws and the bite are misaligned. Above right: multiple abfractions and gum recession sites likely result from teeth grinding.

Uneven facial features are surface indicators of underlying distortion in the cranio-facial skeleton. What can be done in such cases?

A Holistic Mouth doctor needs to possess a wide-ranging knowledge base in order to do their CSI. Sometimes the answer lies outside the traditional medical or dental box. That is the value and the necessity of the WholeHealth mindset – and that is why a Holistic Mouth Doctor is much more than a dentist with a bunch of oral appliances.

If you are a healthcare professional who wants to learn more about CST, visit UpledgerInstitute.com or see the texts listed in the references. [3, 4, 5, 6, 7].

If you are a patient, check out *Your Inner Physician and You* – a great book written for non-health professionals [8] – or visit www.upledger.com/therapies/index.php. [9]

What Jenna's Case Teaches

A doctor's job ideally is the to put the body in a position to heal itself. A powerful way to do this is by facilitating deep sleep through the sleep-airway-mouth connection. The doctors Jenna had seen were the best in their fields, but her body needed help to get Impaired Mouth fixed so sleep and energy can resume through wider airway and better alignment for neurological function.

Is Jenna's case an exception? Yes, but only because every patient is unique. But it is NOT an exception in terms of missing the link of poor sleep, pinched airway, and impaired mouth structure. In principle, the U-turn back to health starts with a three-step process:

> A. Recognizing Impaired Mouth as an anatomical source of many medical, dental, mental and mood symptoms. A medical, dental, or other healthcare degree is not required. Any teachable patient can learn to pick up Liao's Sign and other clues pointing to the mouth as a structural handicap to ABCDES. OneLook YouKnow™ is a program designed

for patients and non-dental health professionals available at www.HolsiticMouthSolutions.com.

B. Realizing that redeveloping an Impaired Mouth into a Holistic Mouth is a natural solution that the body loves. Remember that "Ahhh with a smile" relief that permeates through you when you can breathe through your nose again when you recover from a cold? That's what happens when an Impaired Mouth is restored so the body is "Whole" again.

C. Request a Holistic Mouth checkup by a trained Holistic Mouth doctor to confirm diagnosis and establish a WholeHealth treatment plan that includes or starts with restoring the Sleep-Airway-Mouth link to help make the Whole function naturally again.

Health recovery and maintenance begins with chair side investigation to answer this question: Is your mouth fit to support health?

Recognize your Impaired Mouth, treating it with Holistic Mouth Solutions, and your sleep, mood, and overall health will improve, with facial radiance to show for it.

Holistic Mouth Nuggets

- "How is your sleep?" is the key question in health recovery and wellness maintenance. Chair Side Investigation™ (CSI) begins with the WholeHealth view of the patient. "Is this body getting what it needs to stay health? If not, what's in the way?"

- Cranio-sacral rhythm is as basic to health as sleep and airway. Cranio-sacral therapy provides the right cranial structure for the nervous system in the head to work effectively.

- Impaired Mouth handicaps the whole body with whole body consequences, for which Holistic Mouth is a natural solution. Consider a Holistic Mouth checkup with a dentist trained Holistic Mouth doctor, or consultation online, when your body has not responded to the healthcare given.

Chapter 18

Your Child's Dental-facial Development: Nutritional Lessons from Pottenger's Cats

Inferior doctors treat disease after it is symptomatic
Mediocre doctors treat disease as it becomes symptomatic
Superior doctors treat disease before it is symptomatic

— Nei Jing, the first Chinese medical text (2600 BCE)

Everybody wants a superior doctor, whether the presenting complaint is snoring, teeth grinding, jaw pain, root-canals, heart attack, failed teeth, implants, or brain fog. When you show up too late, you necessarily make your doctor an inferior one.

When you show up in time, you have a shot a make her/him a mediocre or superior one. This is especially the case with children's dental facial development toward Holistic Mouth. Crowded lower front teeth is often the first clue to parents that something is not right.

Why do so many children grow up with bunched up teeth needing braces? Why do so many adults end up with sleep apnea and Alzheimer's disease nowadays? The work of Dr. Weston A. Price, DDS [1] has been covered briefly in chapter 5. Now let's turn to the cat studies of Dr. Francis Pottenger, MD.

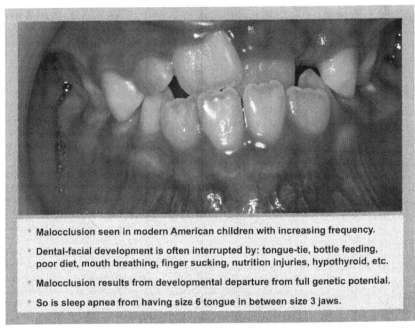

- Malocclusion seen in modern American children with increasing frequency.
- Dental-facial development is often interrupted by: tongue-tie, bottle feeding, poor diet, mouth breathing, finger sucking, nutrition injuries, hypothyroid, etc.
- Malocclusion results from developmental departure from full genetic potential.
- So is sleep apnea from having size 6 tongue in between size 3 jaws.

This 8-year-old may have ancestors who have been on processed for generations.

Poor dental-facial development is "one of the earliest defects noticed in the cats on cooked food.... If proper nutrition and exercise are absent when facial structures are developing, dentition always suffers. The kitten kept on a deficient diet for 10 months has an inadequate jaw with crowded, irregular and poorly aligned teeth." [1]

Dr. Pottenger's studies also showed that nutritional injuries can be passed down from one generation to the next with increasing severity.

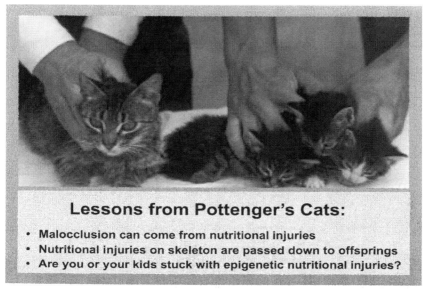

Lessons from Pottenger's Cats:
* **Malocclusion can come from nutritional injuries**
* **Nutritional injuries on skeleton are passed down to offsprings**
* **Are you or your kids stuck with epigenetic nutritional injuries?**

Kittens that cannot run for their lives are not fit to survive in the wild. These came from mother cats fed cooked meat (processed food).

It's Not Your Fault, Mom

A look of concern often show up on the faces of mothers who bring their children to see me. To them I say: do not feel guilty that your child does not have perfectly straight teeth. You should feel great to have found Holistic Mouth as a natural solution.

There are many factors, some of which are beyond your control, while others are. You are responsible only for what's in your control. Now let's look at one that's not.

Is your child on the receiving end of nutritional injuries from up the family tree? And you? Pottenger's Cats have lessons for all parents and doctors. The good news: early intervention to properly develop your child's jaws can fit your child's teeth back into the WholeHealth puzzle.

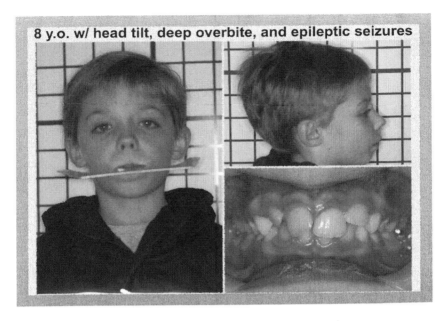

8 y.o. w/ head tilt, deep overbite, and epileptic seizures

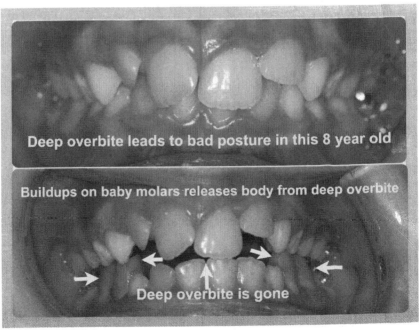

Deep overbite leads to bad posture in this 8 year old

Buildups on baby molars releases body from deep overbite

Deep overbite is gone

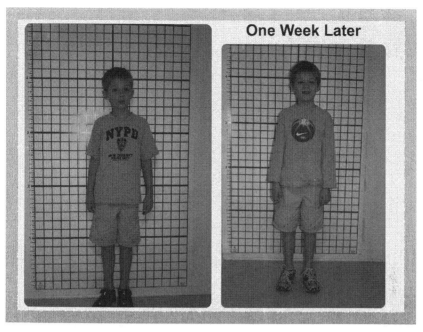

One Week Later

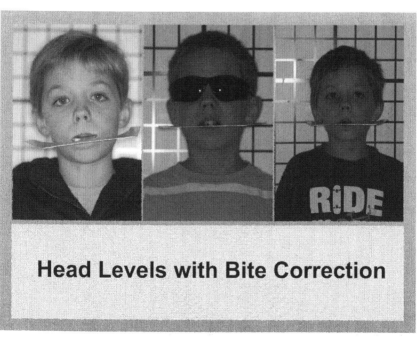

Head Levels with Bite Correction

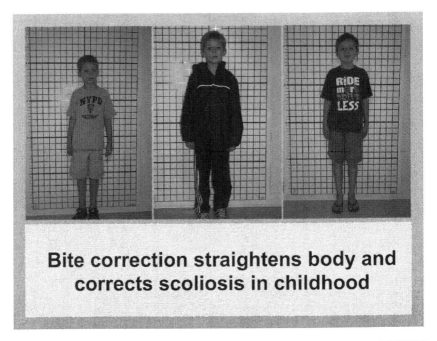

Bite correction straightens body and corrects scoliosis in childhood

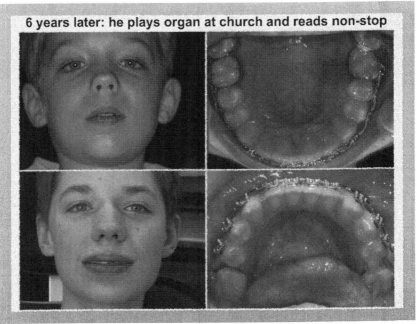

6 years later: he plays organ at church and reads non-stop

This young man has *been free of seizure and medication for 5 years, mainly from diet change and Holistic Mouth development.*

Lessons from Pottenger's Deficient Cats

Dr. Pottenger needed to grow the healthiest cats possible for his research on adrenal glands. By accident, he found the cats on raw meat diet had much more potent adrenals than those on cooked meats prepared for human consumption. If you care about health and wellbeing, you'd sit up and pay intensive attention. So, he studied 2 groups of more than 900 cats over 10 years, and his findings have useful implications for humans.

Both groups were given vitamins, cod liver oil, and given access to outdoors. The control group was fed cat's native diet of raw meat and raw milk. The experimental group was fed a diet of cooked meat and pasteurized milk -- equivalent to processed food for humans. Dr. Pottenger called them Deficient Cats because of the resulting health deficiencies.

"Adults cats placed on cooked meat or pasteurized milk diet begin to show unhealthy condition in their mouths within 3-6 months." [2] Dr. Pottenger's Deficient Cats fed food altered by heat also showed:

- Bad teeth alignment and poor occlusion [3]

- Poor bone mineralization: calcium content of bone ranges from 12-17% in the first deficient generation to 15-30% in the third generation

- Milk produced by a deficient mother lacks the nutrients necessary for her kittens' normal growth and development.

We can infer that if malocclusion leads to weaker adrenals in cats, then it can conceivably lead to weaker everything in humans. Indeed, Dr. Aelred Fonder's has documented malocclusion's oral-systemic complications — see Author's Gift in the Appendix.

The good news: "On the other hand, if such deficient kittens are given adequate feedings during the nursing period, much can be done to improve their general condition." [4]

Raw Meat Group	Cooked Meat Group
Prominent Cheek Bones	Longer and narrower face in Gen2 & 3
Broad Dental Arches	Retruded mid-face, underbite, overbite
Teeth regular in size and alignment	Crowded & Twisted Teeth, Malocclusion
Gregarious, Friendly, Playful	Irritable, nervous, dangerous
Distinct Male & Female Traits	Aggressive females & docile males
Normal sexual interest and pattern	Sexual disinterest or perversion
Strong resistance to parasites	Frequent allergies and skin lesions
Efficient child birth with no delivery complications	25-75% higher aborted pregnancy + difficulty with delivery causing many maternal deaths so there was no 4th generation
Mother cat stays healthy after delivery	Maternal health declines toward death
Newborn average weight = 119 grams	Newborn average weight = 100 grams
Head size stays the same from one gen to the next	Smaller skulls in G2 and G3 kittens
Well-developed normal cat can be maintained in health if given thyroid and adrenals	Does not become a normal cat even if given intense therapy

(Table complied by Dr. Felix Liao, DDS, based on Pottenger's Cats, by Francis Marion Pottenter, Jr., MD, Price-Pottenger Foundation, 1983)

Dr. Pottenger's study reached the same conclusion regarding raw milk compared to to pasteurized milk. "The cats fed pasteurized milk as the principal item of their diet show skeletal changes, lessened reproductive efficiency, and their kittens present progressive constitutional and respiratory problems as is evidenced in the first second and third generation deficient cats eating cooked meat." [5]

Conclusion: processed foods for humans, like cooked meats and pasteurized milk for cats, can result in skeletal injuries that can escalate in successive generations.

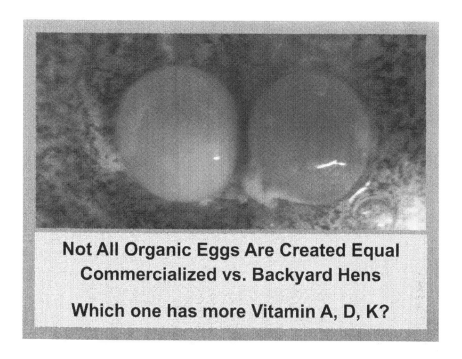

Not All Organic Eggs Are Created Equal
Commercialized vs. Backyard Hens

Which one has more Vitamin A, D, K?

For me, the take-home lessons from Pottenger's Cats are:

A. Some nutrients called "freshness factor" in some foods are heat sensitive.

B. Nutritional injuries, including dental-facial deformities, hormonal imbalances, allergies, and behavioral changes, can come from loss of the "freshness factor"

C. Nutritional injuries first show up in the mouth and dental-facial misalignment

D. Nutritional injuries can be passed down to the next generations to cause increased dental and systemic complications

E. Nutritional injuries and their dental-systemic complications are compounded down the second and third generations, and reversal takes much longer and often is not complete.

Do you have ancestors who had a life time of refined processed foods? Do you have crowded teeth or history of orthodontic braces?

Now you can understand why your child has crowded or crooked teeth.

Knowing WHY gives us a shot at sensible natural solutions. Dr. Pottenger concluded, "The first step in giving a person the right nutrition is to make him able to eat the right foods in sufficient quantify. This depends on the adequacy of his facial development, the strength of his muscles, and the shape of his masticating (chewing) bones."

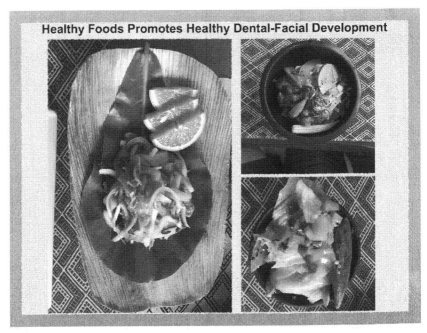

Above: Examples of native Foods from Taiwan's Countryside
Below: Well-formed faces of of Taiwan natives (in red shirts)

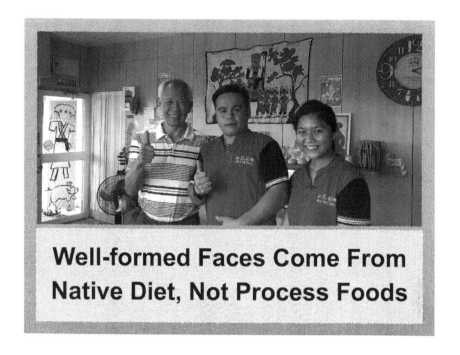

Well-formed Faces Come From Native Diet, Not Process Foods

WholeHealth Kids™: Holistic Mouth Development for Children

Kids may not get to choose parents, but parents can choose what they feed their kids. Diet and family nutritional practices has a profound epigenetic (after-brith) influence of children'd dental-facial development.

WholeHealth Kids™ is my WholeHealth program for guiding parents to participate in their children's dental-facial development toward Holistic Mouth, one that is structurally fit to support ABCDES: alignment, breathing, circulation, digestion, energy, and sleep.

Emmy is now 5 years old, and she has been in my WholeHealth Kids' program since age 2. Her parents initially wanted to avoid cavities for her, and to develop her jaws and face in the direction of Holistic Mouth once they learned of it. They are members of Weston A. Price Foundation (www.WAPF.org) and they have provided Emmy with organic paleo-style and whole food-based Weston Price diet — with no sugar and minimal grains. It's been a great treat watching WholeHealth Kids like Emmy grow up every 6 months.

At Emmy's last checkup, she was bright, curious, energetic, friendly, entertaining, but cooperative when asked. Clinical exam showed that she has had no cavity at all, with ideal arch form in both jaws, and zero nasal obstruction/congestion. I recommended and show Emmy's parents to floss her baby molars after dinner because she's too young to be responsible for a task requiring such high manual dexterity.

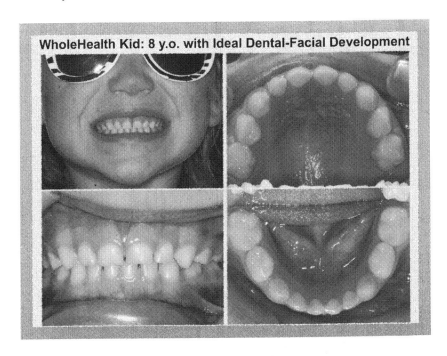

Spacing between front teeth are desirable in children because the replacement adult teeth underneath are bigger than baby teeth. Emmy's upper and lower dental arches indicate sufficient facial skeleton development. No nasal obstruction allows for normal lip seal that is foundational to developing a toward full genetic potential.

Full genetic potential here means having enough jaw volume for all teeth to line up straight naturally with just normal lip and tongue interaction. That's what every human is genetically encoded for, including wisdom teeth. WholeHealth Kids™ guides parents to proactively put their children on Nature's preferred track to Holistic Mouth development.

It's been a great honor and pleasure to work with WholeHealth-minded parents. Emmy's parents have graciously agreed to have her progress photos posted on www.HolsiticMouthSolutions.com, where a free download or Parent's Guide to Children's Holistic Mouth Development is available to help parents and their dentists-turned Holistic Mouth doctors get started in WholeHealth Kids™ program.

You will find a superior doctor every time you go to a Holistic Mouth doctor trained to provide WholeHealth support, whether you are a parent, patient, or healthcare professional.

For More Information
- Read Pottenger's Cats, available from Amazon or Price-Pottenger Nutrition Foundation.
- Join Price-Pottenger Nutrition Foundation, and Weston A. Price Foundation for nutritional tips and classes.
- For individuals and families seeking Holistic Mouth Checkup, please visit www.HolisticMouthSolutions.com.
- Dentists are invited to become a Holistic Mouth doctor: http://holisticmouthsolutions.com/dental/
- Non-dental health professionals are invited to become a Holistic Mouth Consultant: http://holisticmouthsolutions.com/non-dental/

Epilogue

Hearing Early Sirens Leads To Proactive Solutions

Oral diseases and disorders in and of themselves affects health and well-being throughout life.
– David Satcher, MD, PhD,
Oral Health in America: A Report of the Surgeon General
(U.S. Department of Health and Human Services, National
Institute of Dental and Craniofacial Research,
National Institutes of Health, 2000)

This book has shown you how the "scratch the itch" manage-the-symptoms mode of healthcare is outdated because patchwork care doesn't root out the causes.

In contrast, WholeHealth asks, "What does this specific, individual patient need in order to attain sustainable wellbeing? How can the symptoms be traced to their root causes?" The Holistic Mouth approach embodies the WholeHealth logic to create *customized* solutions to make the mouth work for the whole body, and the Whole for the mouth. This requires the attending doctor to have a wide WholeHealth knowledge base beyond the silo of her/his specialty.

What's more, doctors and dentists are just as susceptible to Impaired Mouth Syndrome as their patients. One of dentists taking my training seminars texted this to me: "Just had a really nice internal medical doctor in my chair and she had scoliosis, heart problems, low thyroid, vision problems, crowded lower front teeth, scalloped tongue, dry mouth, uneven shoulders, and lots of root-canals."

I replied, "Thank God you now know how to recognize it and connect the dots to the root cause for her."

As this snapshot and the many cases in this book have shown, a Holistic Mouth is both a proactive prescription for wellness and a natural solution for illness and pain recovery from an Impaired Mouth Syndrome. Very often dramatically crucial.

Financial limitations and lack of health insurance coverage are the major obstacle to starting treatment. Insurers and employers and policy planners can better serve their employees and policy holders with optimal coverage to diagnose and treat the first domino early to head off the costly but avoidable health catastrophes.

By regarding the readily available clues inside and around the mouth indicative of the downhill slide toward sleep apnea, we can stop and reverse your health's decline toward premature aging and poor life quality. By tuning in to the early sirens, we can come up with a proactive solution before it's too late.

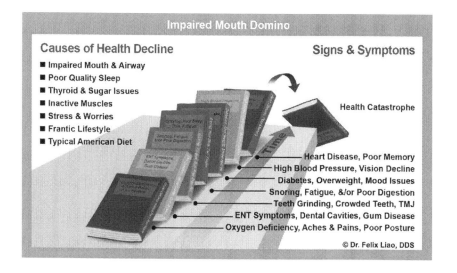

Less Than 1% Know and Can

You now know that there is much more to the Holistic Mouth Solutions than just oral appliance therapy. In fact, if you're a dentist who thinks that training in oral appliance therapy is enough to treat Impaired Mouth Syndrome, think again. According to one company's internal data, only 7% of dentists who take training in oral appliance therapy use it routinely in practice.

Why? Because dentists are trained as tooth doctors, and the vast majority have not been trained in WholeHealth CSI (chair side investigations) in this new era of Oral-Systemic integration, nor Tandem teamwork to best combine oral appliances with other therapies, as needed, for best possible results. Holistic Mouth Solutions offer training seminars to build that WholeHealth diagnostic and collaborative framework.

The mouth is simultaneously dental, medical, social, and an integral part of the Whole. Even if more dentists were to use oral appliances more routinely, jaw orthopedics alone do not heal patients. It takes a wide WholeHealth knowledge base, which is vitally important for all healthcare professionals, not only dentists, to become familiar with Impaired Mouth Syndrome recognition, and Holistic Mouth as a natural solution, regardless of license.

You now understand how undiagnosed Impaired Mouth Syndrome does untold harm, and how Holistic Mouth Solutions™ are crucial far more often than most healthcare professionals, dentists, and patients realize.

What do I mean when I say "most?" In my estimate, less than 1% of dentists currently have a sufficient WholeHealth knowledge base to capably treat Impaired Mouth Syndrome with the cranio-facial orthopedic oral appliances mentioned in this book. The same is likely true of healthcare professionals who know the full picture of Impaired Mouth Domino, and the critical warnings from the mouth regarding health troubles/catastrophes ahead.

Until far more dentists and non-dental healthcare professionals are sufficiently trained in WholeHealth than is currently the case, far too many patients will not find the solutions they're seeking to their dental, medical challenges and natural health quest. It's time to get Impaired Mouth Syndrome and Holistic Mouth Solutions™ on the radar screen of all health professionals.

What's Next for Patients

When your body, or a patient's body, does not respond to the usual treatments for the conditions we've covered in this book, the thing to do next is request a WholeHealth consultation from a qualified specialist, whether in person or online. Make sure it includes a Chair Side Investigation.

If you are a patient or a patient's loved one, and a WholeHealth consultation reveals Impaired Mouth Syndrome, here are two options to consider in deciding what to do next:

- Refer your dentist and healthcare professionals help you by referring them for training seminars in diagnosing Impaired Mouth Syndrome and offering Holistic Mouth Solutions™.

- Seek treatment from a qualified Holistic Mouth doctor.
- Both options are available at www.HolisticMouthSolutions. com and click on "For Individuals & Families".

What's Next for Dentists & Other Healthcare Professionals

- More of your patients will be better served, and you'll end up saving more lives, when you make sure that your patients' airways are evaluated as part of an overall assessment and diagnostic process, and especially if usual treatments aren't working to create recovery or optimal wellness.
- Oral appliances alone do not fix patients. It takes a Holistic Mouth Doctor™ (HMD) with WholeHealth knowledge base and training in oral appliances to connect the dots from symptoms of Impaired Mouth Syndrome to airway, sleep, and a structurally impaired mouth
- Get the information you need, and register for more training, at www.HolisticMouthSolutions.com and click on "For Dental Professionals" or "For Healthcare Professionals".

Got Impaired Mouth? Find Out Your Impaired Mouth Syndrome Score

Is your mouth helping or hurting your health? Is your mouth an asset to your sleep and energy, or a liability? This can be a life-changing question. Finding out your Impaired Mouth Syndrome Score is the place to start finding some answers.

This self-survey begins to illuminate your mouth's structural contributions to medical, dental, and mental-emotional symptoms. It's essentially a checklist of the more common orofacial, dental, and bodily signs and symptoms of impaired mouth. The higher your score, the more likely you have been living with impaired mouth for a long time.

Impaired Mouth Syndrome Score

Mouth	Score	Body	Score
Snoring, morning dry mouth	0 1	Gasping or choking in sleep	0 1
Teeth grinding, jaw	0 1	Neck, shoulder, or back pain; headaches	0 1
Mouth breathing, chapped lips	0 1	Erectile dysfunction or PMS	0 1
Persistent/wandering dental sensitivity	0 1	High blood pressure, heart disease	0 1
Gum recession and/or redness	0 1	Diabetes type 2, bloating after meals	0 1
Clicking/locking jaw joints, zigzag jaw opening	0 1	Weight gain, pot belly; acid reflux	0 1
Morning headache and/or sore jaws	0 1	Daytime sleepiness, fatigue	0 1
Deep overbite or underbite (weak chin)	0 1	Senile memory, ADD/ADHD	0 1
Frequent cavities or broken/chipped teeth	0 1	Frequent colds, flu, and skin disorders	0 1
Teeth prints on the sides of the tongue	0 1	Obstructive sleep apnea from a sleep test	0 1
Bony outgrowth on palate or inside lower jaw	0 1	Stuffy/runny nose, scratchy/itchy throat	0 1
Sunken lips and reverse smile curve (sad)	0 1	Forward head: ears ahead of shoulders	0 1
History of teeth extractions for braces	0 1	Waking up to urinate more than once	0 1
Bulge under lower jaw, double chin	0 1	Large neck size (M>17, W>15)	0 1
History of lots of dental work + medical symptoms	0 1	Poor digestion and elimination	0 1
Malocclusion (crowded teeth)	0 1	Depression, anxiety, grouchiness	0 1
Total Score		Total Score	

www.HolisticMouthSolutions.com

Please note that Impaired Mouth Syndrome Score is not, at this time, a diagnostic tool. No study has been done on it. But it is an excellent conversation starter with your doctor or dentist to rule out impaired mouth. This is how I encourage you to use it – to get the ball rolling so you can get on the path to improved health and vitality through wider airway for deeper sleep.

Holistic Mouth Checkup

The next step is a Holistic Mouth Checkup by a trained health professional, including appropriate imaging of the jaws and oral airway, as well as a sleep test (as needed), to confirm an impaired mouth diagnosis.

A dental checkup covers the teeth and gums, which is an important foundation, of course. A Holistic Mouth Checkup builds on that foundation, by examining the mouth's role in Whole Body health through ABCDES – alignment, breathing, circulation, digestion, energy, and sleep.

To find a properly trained Holistic Mouth Doctor™ near you who can provide you with a Holistic Mouth Checkup, visit HolisticMouthSolutions.com.

Your Daytime Sleepiness: The Epworth Sleepiness Scale

The Epworth Sleepiness Scale is a tool doctors use to evaluate daytime sleepiness – one of the most common signs of sleep apnea and often a clue to airway issues that result from an impaired mouth. This version is commonly used by sleep doctors and sleep researchers, and its originator Dr. Murray Johns has given kind permission to Dr. Liao for its use.

Think about each of the situations listed below, and then rate how likely you are to doze off while engaged in the activities described:

0 = not at all likely to doze
1 = slightly likely
2 = moderately likely
3 = very likely to doze

Situation	Chance of dozing
Sitting & reading	
Watching TV	
Sitting in a public place	
Riding as a passenger in a car for 1 hour	
Lying down in the afternoon	
Sitting & talking with someone	
Sitting quietly after a lunch with no alcohol	
Stopped for a few minutes in traffic	

The average score is 4 to 8. If you score higher than this, you should talk with your doctor – especially if your score is 16 or above.

Please note that the survey presented here is not the official diagnostic tool but is shared as a means of self-assessment, to recognize whether daytime sleepiness is an issue for you so you can seek help as needed from your health care providers.

Dental Distress Syndrome:
Connecting Malocclusion
to Overall Health

Dental stress can be the root or cause of many disorders in the body because it is a constant, unrelenting stress, always operative until the dentist intervenes.

— Aelred C. Fonder, DDS, The Dental Physician [1]

Malocclusion is a big bother to the brain and the whole body. But life must go on, so the body pays a heavy price in terms of chronic and persistent medical symptoms in the presence of stressors.

Dental Distress Syndrome is a term aptly coined by Dr. Fonder to describe malocclusion's effect on overall health. His seminal book by the same title contains many eye-openers. One that really struck me when I first read it was, "low thyroid is almost always a constant finding" in patients with dental bite distress.

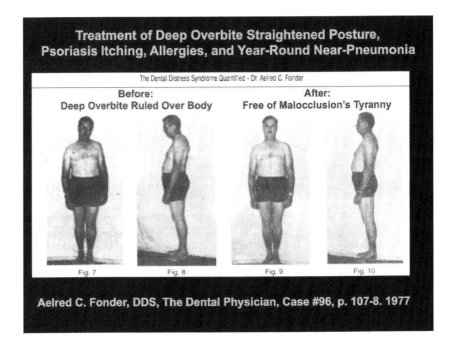

Treatment of Deep Overbite Straightened Posture,
Psoriasis Itching, Allergies, and Year-Round Near-Pneumonia

The Dental Distress Syndrome Quantified - Dr. Aelred C. Fonder

Before:
Deep Overbite Ruled Over Body

After:
Free of Malocclusion's Tyranny

Fig. 7   Fig. 8   Fig. 9   Fig. 10

Aelred C. Fonder, DDS, The Dental Physician, Case #96, p. 107-8. 1977

To read more, please visit
www.HolisticMouthSolutions.com/DentalDistressSyndrome

Holistic Mouth Development: A Parents' Guide

Your child's orofacial and dental development starts well before birth. In the Whole Health approach, a partnership between parents and a doctor of holistic mouth is encouraged, with the following ideals in mind:

Preconception

- Sound and sensible nutrition for 6 to12 months.
- A dental checkup to ensure healthy teeth and sound gums for the mom-to-be.
- A Holistic Mouth Checkup to rule out pinched airway and more.

Immediately After Birth

- Breastfeeding – Nature's way for a baby to develop a wide upper jaw.
- Check for tongue-tie and upper lip-tie if breasts latch is problematic.
- Check for cranial distortion from birth trauma, and seek a cranial osteopathic doctor or craniosacral therapist if crying, irritability, colic, and/or spit-up persist.

To read more, please visit
www.HolsiticMouthSolutions.com/Parents'Guide.

Acknowledgments and Gratitude

I am grateful to all the patients who have contributed to this book with their stories and images, and to all patients who have added to my experience through the years.

I am grateful, too, to all the instructors who have taught me – from dental school to post-graduate seminars in dentistry, medicine, and integrative health, as well as those who have contributed to this book. You know who you are.

I am grateful as well to all the dentists and their staff who have started their training to become Holistic Mouth Doctors™ to diagnose Impaired Mouth Syndrome in their patients and bring Holistic Mouth Solutions™ and WholeHealth Kids™ to their communities.

I thank all my friends and colleagues who have encouraged and supported me through the years of writing this book: Jasmine Ma, Dr. Sharon Fan, Dr. Brendan Stack, Dr. Jay Gerber, Dr. Richard Beistle, Dr. Dennis Bailey, Dr. G. Dave Singh, Dr. Louisa Williams, Dr. George Yu, Dr. Robert Walker, Dr. Je-yang Jau and his graphic artist Jia-Jun Tsai in Taiwan, my editor Lisa Verigin, Sue Glass, Sima Button my graphic artist, Jessie Martin, David Gruder, Linda Kaye, my office staff, my brother Allen, Aunt Grace Lin, all the smart and experienced dental laboratory technicians I've leaned on (you know who you are), Dr. Michaela McKenzie, and Robbin Simons and her superb team at Crescendo Publishing.

About the Author

Dr. Liao is a holistic dentist and mouth doctor devoted to helping patients turn back illness and turn on wellness with Holistic Mouth Solutions. He blends leading edge technology with old-fashioned TLC for children and adults at WholeHealth Dental Center in Falls Church, Virginia.

Dr. Liao's professional mission is to help build whole body health with a holistic mouth — one that is an asset to whole body health rather than a liability. Since dental school, Dr. Liao has been interested in teeth grinding: "Why would the body mutilate the hardest tissue it has?!" Holistic Mouth Solutions result from Dr. Liao's pursuit to find the root cause of teeth grinding and better overall health by mouth.

For patients wishing to cultivate a more holistic mouth style to support overall health, Dr. Liao teaches WholeHealth Wellness Seminars. Dr. Liao also offers Holistic Mouth Seminars to help aspiring dentists and all health professionals to become certified holistic mouth doctors. More information at HolisticMouthSolutions.com.

Dr. Liao is a U.S. citizen born and raised in Taiwan until age 16. He graduated from Brown University with an engineering degree, and Doctor of Dental Surgery from Case School of Dental Medicine. Since dental school, he has taken extensive post-graduate training in integrative medicine, oral-systemic dentistry, nutrition, cranial osteopathy, chiropractics, nutrition, and studies in Traditional Chinese Medicine.

He is a board-certified general dentist with Masterships in both the Academy of General Dentistry and the International Academy of Biological Dentistry and Medicine (IABDM). He is the current president of IABDM.

Dr. Liao has been a speaker at the International College of Integrative Medicine, Weston A. Price Foundation, the Holistic Moms' Network, Take Back Your Health Conference, Academy of Integrative Health and Medicine, and International Academy of Biological Dentistry and Medicine, among others.

Dr. Liao's personal interests includes classical music, organic lifestyle, science, world cuisine and culture, learning and teaching health-building skills, and research connecting cranial-facial-dental development with nutrition and lifestyle habits.

Connect with the Author

Websites: www.HolisticMouthSolutions.com
Email: DrFelix@HolisticMouthSolutions.com

Address: P.O. Box 3325, Merrifield, Virginia 22116
Phone: 703-385-6425

Facebook: https://www.facebook.com/wholehealthdentalcenter/
LinkedIn: https://www.linkedin.com/in/felixliaodds/
Pinterest: https://pinterest.com/wholehealthdentalcenter
Twitter: www.twitter.com/DrFelixLiao
Instagram: HolisticMouthSolutions

Dr. Felix Liao
www.WholeHealthDentalCenter.com
703-385-6425 - Office

References for Early Sirens

Ch.1 Snoring — Health Risks Iceberg Ahead and What Lurks Between and Below

1. William C. Dement and Merrill M. Mitler, "It's Time to Wake Up to the Importance of Sleep Disorders," Journal of the American Medical Association 269, no. 12 (1993): 1548–1550, DOI: 10.1001/jama.1993.03500120086032, PMID: 8445820.

2. Application and approval to market the mRNA appliance, http://www.accessdata.fda.gov/cdrh_docs/pdf13/K130067.pdf.

3. William Beninati and others, "The Effect of Snoring and Obstructive Sleep Apnea on the Sleep Quality of Bed Partners," *Mayo Clinic Proceedings* 74, no. 10 (1999): 955–958, DOI: 10.4065/74.10.955, PMID: 10918859.

4. *M Koskenvuo, J Kaprio, T Telakivi, M Partinen, K Heikkilä,* Snoring as a risk factor for ischemic heart disease and stroke in men. *Br Med J (Clin Res Ed)* 1987;294:16.

5. Eva Lindberg and others, "Evolution of Sleep Apnea Syndrome in Sleepy Snorers," *American Journal of Respiratory and Critical Care Medicine* 159, no. 6 (1999): 2024–2027, DOI: 10.1164/ajrccm.159.6.9805070, PMID: 10351957.

6. Heikki Palomäki, "Snoring and the Risk of Ischemic Brain Infarction," *Stroke* 22, no. 8 (1991): 1021–1025, DOI: 10.1161/01.STR.22.8.1021, PMID: 1866748.

7. J.P. Neau and others, "Habitual Snoring as a Risk Factor for Brain Infarction," *Acta Neurologica Scandinavica* 92, no. 1 (1995): 63–68, DOI: 10.1111/j.1600-0404.1995.tb00468.x, PMID: 7572063.

8. See note 5.

9. Sharon A. Lee and others, "Heavy Snoring as a Cause of Carotid Artery Atherosclerosis," *SLEEP* 31, no. 9 (2008):

1207–1213, http://www.journalsleep.org/ViewAbstract. aspx?pid=27245, PMID: 18788645.

10. Wael K. Al-Delaimy and others, "Snoring as a Risk Factor for Type II Diabetes Mellitus: A Prospective Study," *American Journal of Epidemiology* 155, no. 5 (2002): 387–393, DOI: 10.1093/aje/155.5.387, PMID: 11867347.

11. Dirk Pevernagie, Ronald M. Aarts, and Micheline De Meyer, "The Acoustics of Snoring," *Sleep Medicine Reviews* 14, no. 2 (2010): 131–144, DOI: 10.1016/j. smrv.2009.06.002, PMID: 19665907.

12. E. Lugaresi and others, "Some Epidemiological Data on Snoring and Cardiocirculatory Disturbances," *SLEEP* 3, no. 3 (1980): 221–224, http://www.journalsleep.org/ ViewAbstract.aspx?pid=24221, PMID: 7221330.

13. Wikipedia, Bohr Effect: https://en.wikipedia.org/wiki/ Bohr_effect

14. Ramar K, Dort LC, Katz SG, Lettieri CJ, Harrod CG, Thomas SM, Chervin RD. Clinical practice guideline for the treatment of obstructive sleep apnea and snoring with oral appliance therapy: an update for 2015. J Clin Sleep Med 2015;11(7):773–827.

Ch. 2 The Most Overlooked Key to Health and Performance — Sleep-Airway-Mouth Synergy

1. Dr. Joseph Mercola, "Toxic Food Additives Found in Bread, Pasta Sauce, and Salad Dressing," Mercola. com, March 24, 2012, http://articles.mercola.com/sites/ articles/archive/2012/03/24/hungry-for-change.aspx?e_ cid=20120324_DNL_art_1.

2. Marieke P Hoevenaar-Blom, Annemieke MW Spijkerman, Daan Kromhout and WM Monique Verschuren, Sufficient sleep duration contributes to lower cardiovascular disease risk in addition to four traditional lifestyle factors: the MORGEN study. *European Journal of Preventive Cardiology* 2014, Nov;21(11):1367-75. doi: 10.1177/2047487313493057. Epub 2013 Jul 3. PMID: 23823570

3. Lyndsay Warhead ND, Traditional Chinese Medicine Organ Times:http://www.naturopathicbynature.com/traditional-chinese-medicine-organ-times/

4. Mayo Clinic, Chronic Stress Puts Your Health At Risk. http://www.mayoclinic.org/healthy-lifestyle/stress-management/in-depth/stress/art-20046037

5. Tanja Lange, Stoyan Dimitrov, and Jan Born, "Effects of Sleep and Circadian Rhythm on the Human Immune System," *Annals of the New York Academy of Sciences* 1193 (2010): 48–59, DOI: 10.1111/j.1749-6632.2009.05300.x, PMID: 20398008.

6. F. Javier Nieto and others, "Sleep-Disordered Breathing and Cancer Mortality: Results from the Wisconsin Sleep Cohort Study," *American Journal of Respiratory and Critical Care Medicine* 186, no. 2 (2012): 190–194, DOI: 10.1164/rccm.201201-0130OC, PMID: 22610391.

7. Luca Imeri and Mark R. Opp, "How (and Why) the Immune System Makes Us Sleep," *Nature Reviews Neuroscience* 10 (2009): 199–210, DOI: 10.1038/nrn2576, http://www.ncbi.nlm.nih.gov/pmc/articles/PMC2839418/.

8. Jeannine A. Majde and James M. Krueger, "Links Between the Innate Immune System and Sleep," *Journal of Allergy and Clinical Immunology* 116, no. 6 (2005): 1188–1198, DOI: 10.1016/j.jaci.2005.08.005, PMID: 16337444.

9. Penelope A. Bryant, John Trinder, and Nigel Curtis, "Sick and Tired: Does Sleep Have a Vital Role in the Immune System?" *Nature Reviews Immunology* 4 (2004): 457–467, DOI: 10.1038/nri1369, PMID: 15173834.

10. Allan Rechtschaffen and others, "Sleep Deprivation in the Rat: X. Integration and Discussion of the Findings," *SLEEP* 25, no. 1 (2002): 68–87, http://www.journalsleep.org/ViewAbstract.aspx?pid=25682, PMID: 11833857.

11. David Permitter, MD, with Kristin Loberg, Brain Brain: The Surprising Truth About Wheat, Carbs, and Sugar — Your Brain's Silent Killers. Little, Brown and Company 2013

12. Huang CW, Lui CC, Chang WN, Lu CH, Wang YL, Chang CC. Elevated basal cortisol level predicts lower

hippocampal volume and cognitive decline in Alzheimer's disease. J Clin Neurosci. 2009 Oct;16(10):1283-6. Epub 2009 Jun 30.

13. Anne G. Wheaton and others, "Sleep-Disordered Breathing and Depression Among U.S. Adults: National Health and Nutrition Examination Survey, 2005–2008," *SLEEP* 35, no. 4 (2012): 461–467, DOI: 10.5665/sleep.1724, PMID: 22467983.

14. Centers for Disease Control and Prevention FastStats: http://www.cdc.gov/nchs/fastats/drug-use-therapeutic.htm

15. Emanuela Esposito and Salvatore Cuzzocrea, "Anti-inflammatory Activity of Melatonin in Central Nervous System," *Current Neuropharmacology* 8, no. 3 (2010): 228–242, DOI: 10.2174/157015910792246155, PMID: 21358973.

16. Viktor Roman and others, "Too Little Sleep Gradually Desensitizes the Serotonin 1A Receptor System," *SLEEP* 28, no. 12 (2005): 1505–1510, http://www.journalsleep.org/ViewAbstract.aspx?pid=26275, PMID: 16408408.

17. Mahesh M. Thakkar, "Histamine in the Regulation of Wakefulness," *Sleep Medicine Reviews* 15, no. 1 (2011): 65–74, DOI: 10.1016/j.smrv.2010.06.004, PMID: 20851648.

18. Kaful Dzirasa and others, "Dopaminergic Control of Sleep-Wake States," *Journal of Neuroscience* 26, no. 41 (2006): 10577–10589, DOI: 10.1523/JNEUROSCI.1767-06.2006, PMID: 17035544.

19. Janssen, V., De Gucht, V., Dusseldorp, E., & Maes, S. (2013). Lifestyle Modification Programs for Patients with Coronary Heart Disease: A Systematic Review and Meta-Analysis of Randomiezd Controlled Trials. European Journal of Preventive Cardiology, 20, 620-640. doi:10.1177/204748312462824 (IF=3.04)

Ch. 3 Teeth Grinding — The Inside Story of Sleep Bruxing Airway Disorder

1. Maurice M. Ohayon, Kasey K. Li, and Christian Guilleminault, "Risk Factors for Sleep Bruxism in the

General Population," *Chest* 119, no. 1 (2001): 53–61, DOI: 10.1378/chest.119.1.53, PMID: 11157584.

2. Maria Clotilde Carra, Nelly Huynh, and Gilles J. Lavigne, "Sleep Bruxism: A Comprehensive Overview for the Dental Clinician Interested in Sleep Medicine," *Dental Clinics of North America* 56, no. 2 (2012): 387–413, DOI: 10.1016/j. cden.2012.01.003, PMID: 22480810.

3. See note 1.

4. A. Hachmann and others, "Efficacy of the Nocturnal Bite Plate in the Control of Bruxism for 3 to 5 Year Old Children," *Journal of Clinical Pediatric Dentistry* 24, no. 1 (1999): 9–15, PMID: 10709536.

5. American College of Chest Physicians, "Teeth Grinding Linked to Sleep Apnea; Bruxism Prevalent in Caucasians with Sleep Disorders," *ScienceDaily,* Nov. 5, 2009, http://www.sciencedaily.com/releases/2009/11/091102171213. htm.

6. T.T. Sjöholm and others, "Sleep Bruxism in Patients with Sleep-Disordered Breathing," *Archives of Oral Biology* 45, no. 10 (2000): 889–896, DOI: 10.1016/S0003-9969(00)00044-3, PMID: 10973562.

7. GJ Lavigne, N. Huynh, T. Kato, K. Okura, K. Adachi, D. Yao, B. Sessle, Genesis of sleep bruxism: motor and autonomic-cardiac interactions. Arch Oral Biol. 2007 Apr;52(4):381-4. Epub 2007 Feb 20.

8. Jonathan D. Cogen, John J. Kelly Jr., and Darius A Loghmanee, "Sleep Bruxism," MedMerits, http://www.medmerits.com/index.php/article/sleep_bruxism.

9. See note 2.

10. American College of Chest Physicians, "Teeth Grinding Linked to Sleep Apnea; Bruxism Prevalent in Caucasians with Sleep Disorders," *ScienceDaily,* Nov. 5, 2009, http://www.sciencedaily.com/releases/2009/11/091102171213. htm.

11. T.T. Sjöholm and others, "Sleep Bruxism in Patients with Sleep-Disordered Breathing," *Archives of Oral Biology* 45, no. 10 (2000): 889–896, DOI: 10.1016/S0003-9969(00)00044-3, PMID: 10973562.

12. Angela Nashed and others, "Sleep Bruxism Is Associated with a Rise in Arterial Blood Pressure," *SLEEP* 35, no. 4 (2012): 529–536, DOI: 10.5665/sleep.1740, PMID: 22467991.

13. F. Lobbezoo and others, "Bruxism Defined and Graded: An International Consensus," *Journal of Oral Rehabilitation* 40, no. 1 (2013): 2–4, DOI: 10.1111/joor.12011, PMID: 23121262.

14. American Academy of Sleep Medicine, ed., *International Classification of Sleep Disorders: Diagnostic and Coding Manual,* 2nd ed. (ICSD-2) (Westchester, IL: American Academy of Sleep Medicine, 2005), 189–192.

15. "Teeth Grinding," National Sleep Foundation, https://sleepfoundation.org/sleep-disorders-problems/bruxism-and-sleep.

16. DG Simons, JG Travell, LS Simons, Myofascial Pain and Dysfunction The Trigger Point Manual,1999, Williams & Wilkins.

17. See note 2.

18. "TMJ (TMD) and Sleep Bruxism Associated with OSA: Diagnosis and Treatment Explained by Dr. Simmons," YouTube video, 4:46, posted by Comprehensive Sleep Medicine Associates, July 23, 2011, http://www.youtube.com/watch?v=HKrSIzDyoN4.

19. Gaby G. Bader and others, "Descriptive Physiological Data on a Sleep Bruxism Population," *SLEEP* 20, no. 11 (1997): 982–990, http://www.journalsleep.org/ViewAbstract.aspx?pid=24236, PMID: 9456463,.

20. Gilles J. Lavigne and others, "Genesis of Sleep Bruxism: Motor and Autonomic-Cardiac Interactions," *Archives of Oral Biology* 52, no. 4 (2007): 381–384, DOI: 10.1016/j.archoralbio.2006.11.017, PMID: 17313939.

21. Angela Nashed and others, "Sleep Bruxism Is Associated with a Rise in Arterial Blood Pressure," *SLEEP* 35, no. 4 (2012): 529–536, DOI: 10.5665/sleep.1740, PMID: 22467991.

22. Frank Lobbed and M. Naeije, "Bruxism Is Mainly Regulated Centrally, Not Peripherally," *Journal of Oral*

Rehabilitation 28, no. 12 (2001): 1085–1091, DOI:
10.1046/j.1365-2842.2001.00839.x, PMID: 11874505.

23. See note 2.

Ch. 4 "I Ground Through My Night Guard" — A Holistic Mouth Solutions Case Study

1. Dr. Joseph Mercola, "The Greatest Nutrition Researcher of the 20th Century," Mercola.com, Oct. 6, 2007, http://articles.mercola.com/sites/articles/archive/2007/10/06/the-greatest-nutrition-researcher-of-the-twentieth-century.aspx.

2. G. Dave Singh and James A. Krumholtz, *Epigenetic Orthodontics in Adults* (Chatsworth, CA: Smile Foundation, 2009), 26.

3. Xavier Barceló and others, "Oropharyngeal Examination to Predict Sleep Apnea Severity," *Archives of Otolaryngology — Head & Neck Surgery* 137, no. 10 (2011): 990–996, DOI: 10.1001/archoto.2011.176, PMID: 22006776.

4. Sally Fallon, Nourishing Traditions Diet. New Trends Publishing (2003) 2nd edition.

5. Dr. Joseph Marcela, How the Buteyko Breathing Method Can Improve Your Health and Fitness

6. Academy of Orofacial Myofunctional Therapy, "Frequently Asked Questions and Answers in the Area of Orofacial Myofunctional Therapy" (Pacific Palisades, CA: Academy of Orofacial Myofunctional Therapy, 2014).

7. Patrick McKeown, Close Your Mouth: Stop Asthma, Hay Fever, and Nasal Congestion Permanently. Buteyko Books, Galway 2004.

8. Felix Liao and G. Dave Singh, "Resolution of Sleep Bruxism Using Biomimetic Oral Appliance Therapy: A Case Report," *Journal of Sleep Disorders & Therapy* 4, no. 4 (2015), DOI: 10.4172/2167-0277.1000204.

Ch. 5 Holistic Mouth Epigenetics — Harnessing Your Stem Cells to Put Your Best Face Forward

1. Yosh Jefferson, "Facial Beauty — Establishing a Universal Standard," *International Journal of Orthodontics* 15, no. 1 (2004), 9–22, http://www.facialbeauty.org/article/FacialBeauty.pdf.

2. "What Is the Difference Between Epigenetics and Epigenomics?" Epigenesys, http://www.epigenesys.eu/it/public/faq-common/111-what-is-the-difference-between-epigenetics-and-epigenomics.

3. Yosh Jefferson, "Mouth Breathing: Adverse Effects on Facial Growth, Health, Academics, and Behavior," *General Dentistry* 58, no. 1 (2010): 18–25, PMID: 20129889, http://www.jeffersondental.com/assets/docs/mouthBreathing.pdf.

4. "Epigenomics," National Human Genome Research Institute, http://www.genome.gov/27532724.

5. Weston A. Price, *Nutrition and Physical Degeneration* (Lemon Grove, CA: Price-Pottenger Nutrition Foundation, 2008). An earlier version of the book can be read at http://gutenberg.net.au/ebooks02/0200251h.html or http://journeytoforever.org/farm_library/price/pricetoc.html.

6. Francis M. Pottenger Jr., *Pottenger's Cats: A Study in Nutrition,* 2nd ed. (Lemon Grove, CA: Price-Pottenger Nutrition Foundation, 1995).

7. Epigenomics," National Human Genome Research Institute, https://www.genome.gov/27532724Epigenome Fact Sheet.

8. Sally Fallon, Nourishing Traditions Diet. New Trends Publishing (2003) 2nd edition.

9. Dr. Joseph Marcela, How the Buteyko Breathing Method Can Improve Your Health and Fitness

10. G. Dave Singh and James A. Krumholtz, *Epigenetic Orthodontics in Adults* (Chatsworth, CA: Smile Foundation, 2009).

11. Trish E. Parsons and others, "Mind the Gap: Genetic Manipulation of Basicranial Growth Within Synchondroses Modulates Calvarial and Facial Shape in Mice Through

Epigenetic Interactions," *PLOS ONE* 10, no. 2 (2015): e0118355, DOI: 10.1371/journal.pone.0118355, PMID: 25692674.

12. "What Is the Epigenome?" in *Genetics Home Reference: Your Guide to Understanding Genetic Conditions* (Bethesda, MD: Lister Hill National Center for Biomedical Communications, U.S. National Library of Medicine, National Institutes of Health, Department of Health & Human Services, 2015), http://ghr.nlm.nih.gov/handbook/howgeneswork/epigenome.

13. G. Dave Singh, email message to author, Dec. 7, 2015.

Ch. 6   Impaired Mouth Treated and Untreated — A Tale of Two Brothers' Cases

1.   Jonathan E. Shaw and others, "Sleep-Disordered Breathing and Type 2 Diabetes: A Report from the International Diabetes Federation Taskforce on Epidemiology and Prevention," *Diabetes Research and Clinical Practice* 81, no. 1 (2008): 2–12, DOI: 10.1016/j.diabres.2008.04.025, PMID: 18544448, http://www.idf.org/webdata/docs/DRCP%2081%281%29%20Shaw%20et%20al.pdf.

2.   G. Dave Singh, "Guest Editorial on the Etiology and Significance of Palatal and Mandibular Tori," *CRANIO: The Journal of Craniomandibular & Sleep Practice* 28, no. 4 (2010): 213–215, DOI: 10.1179/crn.2010.030, PMID: 21032973.

3.   "Sleep Apnoea and Type 2 Diabetes," International Diabetes Federation, http://www.idf.org/sleep-apnoea-and-type-2-diabetes; N. Meslier and others, "Impaired Glucose-Insulin Metabolism in Males with Obstructive Sleep Apnea Syndrome," *European Respiratory Journal* 22, no. 1 (2003): 156–160, DOI: 10.1183/09031936.03.00089902, PMID: 12882466.

4.   "Sleep Apnoea and Type 2 Diabetes," International Diabetes Federation, http://www.idf.org/sleep-apnoea-and-type-2-diabetes; S.D. West, D.J. Nicoll, and J.R. Stradling, "Prevalence of Obstructive Sleep Apnea in Men with Type

2 Diabetes," *Thorax* 61, no.11 (2006): 945–950, DOI: 10.1136/thx.2005.057745, PMID: 16928713.

5. "Sleep Apnoea and Type 2 Diabetes," International Diabetes Federation, http://www.idf.org/sleep-apnoea-and-type-2-diabetes; Helaine E. Resnick and others, "Diabetes and Sleep Disturbances: Findings from the Sleep Heart Health Study," *Diabetes Care* 26, no. 3 (2003): 702–709, DOI: 10.2337/diacare.26.3.702, PMID: 12610025.

Ch. 7   What Color is Your Airway? Linking Acid Reflux, Sensitive Teeth, Impaired Mouth

1. Steven Y. Park, MD, How Sleep Apnea Causes Pepsin Reflux: http://doctorstevenpark.com/how-sleep-apnea-causes-pepsin-reflux.P.

2. GERD and Sleep, National Science Foundation.org.

3. Demeter, A. Pap, The relationship between gastroesophageal reflux disease and obstructive sleep apnea. J Gastroenterol. 2004 Sep;39(9):815-20.

4. See note 2

5. See note 3

6. Yasuhiro Fujiwara, Tetsuo Arakawa, Ronnie Fass, Gastroesophageal reflux disease and sleep disturbances, J Gastroenterol. 2012 Jul;47(7):760–9.

7. Hye-kyung Jung, M.D., Rok Seon Choung, M.D., and Nicholas J. Talley, M.D., Ph.D., Gastroesophageal Reflux Disease and Sleep Disorders: Evidence for a Causal Link and Therapeutic Implications. J Neurogastroenterol Motil. 2010 Jan; 16(1): 22–29. doi: 10.5056/jnm.2010.16.1.22

8. Anna Lindam, Bradley J. Kendall, Aaron P. Thrift, Graeme A. Macdonald, Suzanne O'Brien, Jesper Lagergren, and David C. Whiteman, Symptoms of Obstructive Sleep Apnea, Gastroesophageal Reflux and the Risk of Barrett's Esophagus in a Population-Based Case-Control Study, PLoS One. 2015; 10(6): e0129836. doi: 10.1371/journal.pone.0129836. PMCID: PMC4474428.

Ch. 8 You Too Can Be "Very Happy I Didn't Need Another Root-canal!"

1. DJ Caplan, et al, The relationship between self-reported history of endodontic therapy and coronary heart disease in the Atherosclerosis Risk in Communities Study. J Am Dent Assoc. 2009 Aug;140(8):1004-12. PMID: 19654253

2. Josef Issels, MD, Cancer A Second Opinion: The Classic Book on Integrative Cancer Treatment, Square One Publishers 2005

3. Joseph Marcela, Why You Should Avoid Root Canals Like A Plague: http://articles.mercola.com/sites/articles/archive/2010/11/16/why-you-should-avoid-root-canals-like-the-plague.aspx

4. Robert Kulacz DDS and Thomas E. Levy, MD, JD. The Toxic Teeth: How a root-canal could be making you sick. MedFox Publishing 2014

5. George E. Meinig, Root Canal Cover Up

6. Thomas Levy, MD, JD, Hidden Epidemic: Silent Oral Infections Cause Most Heart Attacks and Breast Cancers, MedFox Publishing, Henderson Nevada 2017.

7. James Wolcott, DDS, John Meyers, DDS, Endodontic Retreatment or Implants: A Contemporary Conundrum. American Association of Endodontists. https://www.aae.org/uploadedfiles/clinical_resources/wolcott.pdf

8. Louisa Williams, DC, ND, The importance of Acute Supportive Care in Biological Dentistry: http://journal.iabdm.org/the-importance-of-acute-supportive-care-in-biological-dentistry/

9. Pessi T, et al, Bacterial Signatures in Thrombus Aspirates of Patients with Myocardial Infarction, *Circulation*. 2013;127:1219-1228.

10. ADA Council on Scientific Affairs. Dental endosseous implants: an update. J Am Dent Assoc. 2004;135:92-97.

11. Jerry Tennant, MD, Healing Is Voltage, 2013.

12. Giovanni Mariocia, The Foundations of Chinese Medicine, Elsevier Health Sciences, 2005. P. 100.

13. Yubin Lu, Chengcai Lui, Concepts and Theories of Traditional Chinese Medicine. Wiley & Sons, 1998. P.172

14. David G. Simons, Janet G. Travell, and Lois S. Simons, Myofascial Pain and Dysfunction: The Trigger Point Manual, vol. 1, Upper Half of Body, 2nd ed. (Baltimore, MD: Lippincott Williams & Wilkins, 1998).

15. Jenkelson Robert R, Neuromuscular Dental Diagnosis and Treatment, 1990. Ishiyaku EuroAmerica, Inc. Publishers.

Ch. 9 WholeHealth Care — Putting Common Sense Back into Medical and Dental Practices

1. Bradley Bale and Amy Doneen, "Chapter 3: Red Flags — Are You at Risk?" in *Beat The Heart Attack Gene: The Revolutionary Plan to Prevent Heart Disease, Stroke, and Diabetes* (Nashville, TN: Turner Publishing Company, 2014), 43–44.

2. Tanja Pessi and others, "Bacterial Signatures in Thrombus Aspirates of Patients with Myocardial Infarction," *Circulation* 127 (2013): 1219–1228, DOI: 10.1161/CIRCULATIONAHA.112.001254, PMID: 23418311.

3. Mikko J. Pyysalo and others, "The Connection Between Ruptured Cerebral Aneurysms and Odontogenic Bacteria," *Journal of Neurology, Neurosurgery, and Psychiatry* 84, no. 11 (2013): 1214 –1218, DOI: 10.1136/jnnp-2012-304635.

4. Takahiro Ohki and others, "Detection of Periodontal Bacteria in Thrombi of Patients with Acute Myocardial Infarction by Polymerase Chain Reaction," American Heart Journal 163, no. 2 (2012): 164–167, DOI: 10.1016/j.ahj.2011.10.012, PMID: 22305832.

5. Moise Desvarieux and others, "Periodontal Bacteria and Hypertension: The Oral Infections and Vascular Disease Epidemiology Study (INVEST)," Journal of Hypertension 28, no. 7 (2010): 1413–1421, DOI: 10.1097/HJH.0b013e328338cd36, PMID: 20453665.

Ch. 10 Hidden Heart Attack Risk Revealed by Holistic Mouth Checkup: CSI of S.G.

1. Felix Liao, "Is Your Sleep Partner at Risk for a Heart Attack?" Holistic Mouth Doctor Blog, Sept. 11, 2013, http://wholehealthdentalcenter.com/1283/is-your-sleep-partner-at-risk-for-heart-attack/.

2. "Leading Causes of Death," Centers for Disease Control and Prevention, http://www.cdc.gov/nchs/fastats/leading-causes-of-death.htm.

3. William C. Dement and Merrill M. Mitler, "It's Time to Wake Up to the Importance of Sleep Disorders," Journal of the American Medical Association 269, no. 12 (1993): 1548–1550, DOI: 10.1001/jama.1993.03500120086032, PMID: 8445820.

4. Society for Heart Attack Prevention and Eradication, http://www.shapesociety.org/.

5. Marieke P Hoevenaar-Blom, Annemieke MW Spijkerman, Daan Kromhout and WM Monique Verschuren, Sufficient sleep duration contributes to lower cardiovascular disease risk in addition to four traditional lifestyle factors: the MORGEN study. *European Journal of Preventive Cardiology* published online 3 July 2013 DOI: 10.1177/2047487313493057.

6. Moise Desvarieux and others, "Periodontal Bacteria and Hypertension: The Oral Infections and Vascular Disease Epidemiology Study (INVEST)," Journal of Hypertension 28, no. 7 (2010): 1413–1421, DOI: 10.1097/HJH.0b013e328338cd36, PMID: 20453665.

7. International Academy of Biological Dentistry & Medicine: www.IABDM.org

8. Felix K. Liao, DDS, *Six-Foot Tiger Three-Foot Cage,* Crescendo Publishing, 2017

9. Xavier Barceló and others, "Oropharyngeal Examination to Predict Sleep Apnea Severity," *Archives of Otolaryngology — Head & Neck Surgery* 137, no. 10 (2011): 990–996, DOI: 10.1001/archoto.2011.176, PMID: 22006776.

10. G. Dave Singh, "Guest Editorial on the Etiology and Significance of Palatal and Mandibular Tori," CRANIO: The Journal of Craniomandibular & Sleep Practice 28, no. 4 (2010): 213–215, PMID: 21032973, http://www.smileprofessionals.com/uploads/Cranio-2010-Tori-Singh.pdf.

11. Reyes Enciso and others, "Comparison of CBCT Parameters and Sleep Questionnaires in Sleep Apnea Patients and Control Subjects," *Oral Surgery, Oral Medicine, Oral Pathology, Oral Radiology, and Endodontology* 109, no. 2 (2010): 285–293, DOI: 10.1016/j.tripleo.2009.09.033, PMID: 20123412.

12. Gaby G. Bader and others, "Descriptive Physiological Data on a Sleep Bruxism Population," SLEEP 20, no. 11 (1997): 982–990, http://www.journalsleep.org/ViewAbstract.aspx?pid=24236, PMID: 9456463.

13. Angela Nashed and others, "Sleep Bruxism Is Associated with a Rise in Arterial Blood Pressure," SLEEP 35, no. 4 (2012): 529–536, DOI: 10.5665/sleep.1740, PMID: 22467991.

14. Takahiro Ohki and others, "Detection of Periodontal Bacteria in Thrombi of Patients with Acute Myocardial Infarction by Polymerase Chain Reaction," American Heart Journal 163, no. 2 (2012): 164–167, DOI: 10.1016/j.ahj.2011.10.012, PMID: 22305832.

15. Moise Desvarieux and others, "Periodontal Bacteria and Hypertension: The Oral Infections and Vascular Disease Epidemiology Study (INVEST)," Journal of Hypertension 28, no. 7 (2010): 1413–1421, DOI: 10.1097/HJH.0b013e328338cd36, PMID: 20453665.

16. T.T. Sjöholm and others, "Sleep Bruxism in Patients with Sleep-Disordered Breathing," Archives of Oral Biology 45, no. 10 (2000): 889–896, DOI: 10.1016/S0003-9969(00)00044-3, PMID: 10973562.

17. American College of Chest Physicians, "Teeth Grinding Linked to Sleep Apnea; Bruxism Prevalent in Caucasians with Sleep Disorders," ScienceDaily, Nov. 5, 2009, http://www.sciencedaily.com/releases/2009/11/091102171213.htm.

18. Maurice M. Ohayon, Kasey K. Li, and Christian Guilleminault, "Risk Factors for Sleep Bruxism in the General Population," Chest 119, no. 1 (2001): 53–61, DOI: 10.1378/chest.119.1.53, PMID: 11157584.

19. Arie Oksenberg and Elena Arons, "Sleep Bruxism Related to Obstructive Sleep Apnea: The Effect of Continuous Positive Airway Pressure," Sleep Medicine 3, no. 6 (2002): 513–515, DOI: 10.1016/S1389-9457(02)00130-2, PMID: 14592147.

20. Jo-Dee L. Lattimore, David S. Celermajer, and Ian Wilcox, "Obstructive Sleep Apnea and Cardiovascular Disease," *Journal of the American College of Cardiology* 41, no. 9 (2003): 1429–1437, DOI: 10.1016/S0735-1097(03)00184-0, PMID: 12742277.

21. Toshihide Watanabe and others, "Contribution of Body Habitus and Craniofacial Characteristics to Segmental Closing Pressures of the Passive Pharynx in Patients with Sleep-Disordered Breathing," American Journal of Respiratory and Critical Care Medicine 165, no. 2 (2002): 260–265, DOI: 10.1164/ajrccm.165.2.2009032, PMID: 11790665.

22. T. Douglas Bradley and others, "Pharyngeal Size in Snorers, Nonsnorers, and Patients with Obstructive Sleep Apnea," New England Journal of Medicine 315, no. 21 (1986): 1327–1331, DOI: 10.1056/NEJM198611203152105, PMID: 3773955.

23. Germaine Loo and others, "Prognostic Implication of Obstructive Sleep Apnea Diagnosed by Post-Discharge Sleep Study in Patients Presenting with Acute Coronary Syndrome," Sleep Medicine 15, no. 6 (2014): 631–636, DOI: 10.1016/j.sleep.2014.02.009, PMID: 24796286.

Ch. 11 Dental Angina – Successful WholeHealth Rescue of Qualified Toothaches

1. Mayo Clinic, Angina Definition: http://www.mayoclinic.org/diseases-conditions/angina/basics/definition/con-20031194.

2. Loui WS, et al, Obstructive sleep apnea manifesting as suspected angina: report of three cases. Mayo Clin Proc. 1994 Mar;69(3):244-8. PMID: 8133662.

3. Chan HS, et al, Obstructive sleep apnea presenting with nocturnal angina, heart failure, and near-miss sudden death. Chest. 1991 Apr;99(4):1023-5. PMID: 2009755

4. J T Dodge, B G Brown, E L Bolson, H T Dodge. Lumen diameter of normal human coronary arteries. Influence of age, sex, anatomic variation, and left ventricular hypertrophy or dilation. *Circulation 1992;* 86:232-241. https://doi.org/10.1161/01.CIR.86.1.232.

5. Martos J, Tatsch GH, Tatsch AC, Silveira LF, Ferrer-Luque CM. Anatomical evaluation of the root-canal diameter and root thickness on the apical third of mesial roots of molars. Anat Sci Int. 2011 Sep;86(3):146-50. doi: 10.1007/s12565-011-0102-1. Epub 2011 Mar 17.

6. Akira Tamura MD, et al,   Association between coronary spastic angina pectoris and obstructive sleep apnea. J. Cardiology, September 2010 Volume 56, Issue 2, Pages 240–244. DOI: http://dx.doi.org/10.1016/j.jjcc.2010.06.003

7. Ohki T1, Itabashi Y, Kohno T, Yoshizawa A, Nishikubo S, Watanabe S, Yamane G, Ishihara K. Detection of periodontal bacteria in thrombi of patients with acute myocardial infarction by polymerase chain reaction. Am Heart J. 2012 Feb;163(2):164-7. doi: 10.1016/j.ahj.2011.10.012. PMID: 22305832 DOI: 10.1016/j.ahj.2011.10.012

8. Robert R. Jenkelson, Neuromuscular Dental Diagnosis and Treatment, 1990, p. 33 Ishiyaku EuroAmerica, Inc. Publishers.

9. Robert R. Jenkelson, Neuromuscular Dental Diagnosis and Treatment, 1990, p. 35 Ishiyaku EuroAmerica, Inc. Publishers.

10. David G. Simons, Janet G. Travell, and Lois S. Simons, Myofascial Pain and Dysfunction: The Trigger Point Manual, vol. 1, Upper Half of Body, 2nd ed. P. 279 + 292. (Baltimore, MD: Lippincott Williams & Wilkins, 1998).

11. Robert R. Jenkelson, Neuromuscular Dental Diagnosis and Treatment, 1990, p. 38 Ishiyaku EuroAmerica, Inc. Publishers.

Ch. 12 The Tyranny of Malocclusion — Pain, Fatigue, and Many Surprising Nasty Side Effects

1. Smioka T, Systemic Effects of the Peripheral Effects of the Trigeminal System: Influence of the Occlusal Destruction in Dogs, J. Kyoto Pref. Univ. Med. 98(10) 1077-1085,1989.

2. Profitt WR, et al, Int J Adult Orthodon Orthognath Surg. 198;13(2):97-106. PMID: 9743642

3. Jenkelson Robert R, Neuromuscular Dental Diagnosis and Treatment, 1990. P. 34. Ishiyaku EuroAmerica, Inc. Publishers.

4. Robert M. Sapolsky, Why Zebras Don't Get Ulcers. 3rd ed., Henry Holt and Company 2004.

5. David G. Simons, Janet G. Travell, and Lois S. Simons, Myofascial Pain and Dysfunction: The Trigger Point Manual, vol. 1, Upper Half of Body, p. 178. 2nd ed. (Baltimore, MD, Lippincott Williams & Wilkins, 1998).

6. Jenkelson Robert R, Neuromuscular Dental Diagnosis and Treatment, 1990. P. 37-40. Ishiyaku EuroAmerica, Inc. Publishers.

Ch. 13 "Thank you for giving my wife back to me, Doc." — A Primer on TMJ Pain & Dysfunction

1. Singh GD, et al, Case report: Effect of mandibular tori removal on obstructive sleep apnea parameters. Dialogue, 1, 22-24, 2012.

2. Robert R. Jenkelson, Neuromuscular Dental Diagnosis and Treatment, 1990, p. 35 Ishiyaku EuroAmerica, Inc. Publishers.

3. Robert R. Jenkelson, Neuromuscular Dental Diagnosis and Treatment, 1990, p. 32 Ishiyaku EuroAmerica, Inc. Publishers.

4. Fuentes MA, et al, Lateral functional shift of the mandible: Part II. Effects on gene expression in condylar cartilage. Am J Orthodontics and Dentofacial Orthopedics 2003;123:160-6.

5. Robert R. Jenkelson, Neuromuscular Dental Diagnosis and Treatment, 1990, p. 69 Ishiyaku EuroAmerica, Inc. Publishers.

6. Robert R. Jenkelson, Neuromuscular Dental Diagnosis and Treatment, 1990, p. 12 Ishiyaku EuroAmerica, Inc. Publishers.

7. Jay W. Gerber, DDS, TRMD Warning Sings: Cephalometrics. The functional Orthodontist, march/april 1994, p. 14-19.

8. Chris Chapman, DC, G. Dave Singh, DDSc, PhD, Combined Effect of BioMimetic Oral Appliance and Atlas Orthogonist Cervical Adjustments on Leg Lengths in Adults. A. Vertebral Subluxation Res. August 15, 2013

9. Patrick McKeown, Close Your Mouth: Stop Asthma, Hay Fever, and Nasal Congestion Permanently. Buteyko Books, Galway 2004.

10. Academy of Orofacial Myofunctional Therapy, Myofunctional Therapy and Sleep Disorders: Critical New Research.

11. John E. Upledger, D,O, O.M.M., CranioSacral Therapy, Touchstone for Natural Health and SomotoEmotional Release, 2004. UI Enterprises, Florida.

Ch. 14 Back Pain and Jaw Pain Go Poof — How Root Causes Are Found and Treated in 3 Case Studies

1. No references to note

Ch. 15 Airway First: Find and Fix It Before Dental Implants and Reconstruction

1. Fonders AC, The Dental Physician, second revised edition, Medical-Dental Arts Press, p. 152.

2. Chrcanovic BR, Kisch J, Albrektsson T, Wennerberg A. Bruxism and dental implant failures: a multilevel mixed effects parametric survival analysis approach.J Oral Rehabil. 2016 Nov;43(11):813-823. doi: 10.1111/joor.12431. Epub 2016 Sep 9. PMID: 27611304

3. Quirynen M, Naert I, Van Steenberghe D. Fixture design and overload influence marginal bone loss and fixture success in the Branemark system. Clin Oral Implants Res. 1992;113:104-111.

4. Linish Vidyasagar, Peteris Apse, Dental Implant Design and Biological Effects on Bone-Implant Interface. Stomatologija, Baltic Dental and Maxillofacial Journal, 6:51-4, 2004

5. See note 1.

6. Angela Nashed and others, "Sleep Bruxism Is Associated with a Rise in Arterial Blood Pressure," SLEEP 35, no. 4 (2012): 529–536, DOI: 10.5665/sleep.1740, PMID: 22467991.

7. T.T. Sjöholm and others, "Sleep Bruxism in Patients with Sleep-Disordered Breathing," Archives of Oral Biology 45, no. 10 (2000): 889–896, DOI: 10.1016/S0003-9969(00)00044-3, PMID: 10973562.

8. Shyam Subramanian et al, American College of Chest Physicians, "Teeth Grinding Linked to Sleep Apnea; Bruxism Prevalent in Caucasians with Sleep Disorders," ScienceDaily, Nov. 5, 2009, http://www.sciencedaily.com/releases/2009/11/091102171213.htm.

9. Arie Oksenberg and Elena Arons, "Sleep Bruxism Related to Obstructive Sleep Apnea: The Effect of Continuous Positive Airway Pressure," Sleep Medicine 3, no. 6 (2002): 513–515, DOI: 10.1016/S1389-9457(02)00130-2, PMID: 14592147.

10. Michael Gelb, DDS, Airway Centric Paradigm. CDA Journal, Vol 42, No.8, August 2014.

Ch. 16 Impaired Brain from Impaired Mouth: a Proactive WholeHealth strategy

1. Miles O'Brien and Ann Kellan, "The Connection Between Memory and Sleep," *Science Nation,* Jan. 14, 2013, http://www.nsf.gov/news/special_reports/science_nation/sleepmemory.jsp.

2. Dementia is the Most Costly Disease in America, Alzheimer's Association: http://act.alz.org/site/MessageViewer?dlv_id=101541&em_id=80007.0

3. U.S. Centers for Disease Control and Prevention FastStats: http://www.cdc.gov/nchs/fastats/leading-causes-of-death.htm

4. Mark T McAuley, Rose Anne Kenny, Thomas BL Kirkwood, Darren J Wilkinson, Janette JL Jones and Veronica M Miller. A mathematical model of aging-related and cortisol induced hippocampal dysfunction. BMC Neuroscience2009**10**:26. DOI: 10.1186/1471-2202-10-26

5. Chi-Wei Huang, Chun-Chung Lui, Weng-Neng Chang, Cheng-Hsien Lu, Ya-Ling Wang, Chiung-Chih Chang, Elevated basal cortisol level predicts lower hippocampal volume and cognitive decline in Alzheimer's disease. J. Clinical Neuroscience, October 2009, Volume 16, Issue 10, 1283-1286. DOI: http://dx.doi.org/10.1016/j.jocn.2008.12.026

6. See Note 3.

7. Lois M. Collins, "Treating Sleep Apnea May Head Off Alzheimer's, Other Dementia," *Deseret News,* Aug. 24, 2011, http://www.deseretnews.com/article/700173212/Treating-sleep-apnea-may-head-off-Alzheimers-other-dementia.html?pg=1.

8. Kristine Yaffe and others, "Sleep-Disordered Breathing, Hypoxia, and Risk of Mild Cognitive Impairment and Dementia in Older Women," *Journal of the American Medical Association* 306, no. 6 (2011): 613–619, DOI: 10.1001/jama.2011.1115, PMID: 21828324.

9. See Note 4.

10. Jana R. Cooke and others, "Sustained Use of CPAP Slows Deterioration of Cognition, Sleep, and Mood in Patients with Alzheimer's Disease and Obstructive Sleep Apnea: A Preliminary Study," *Journal of Clinical Sleep Medicine* 5, no. 4 (2009): 305–309, http://www.aasmnet.org/jcsm/ViewAbstract.aspx?pid=27538, PMID: 19968005.

11. Sonia Ascoli-Israel and others, "Cognitive Effects of Treating Obstructive Sleep Apnea in Alzheimer's Disease: A Randomized Controlled Study," *Journal of the American Geriatrics Society* 56, no. 11 (2008): 2076–2081, DOI: 10.1111/j.1532-5415.2008.01934.x, PMID: 18795985.

12. W.H. Seo and others, "The Association Between Periodontitis and Obstructive Sleep Apnea: A Preliminary Study," *Journal of Periodontal Research* 48, no. 4 (2013): 500–506, DOI: 10.1111/jre.12032, PMID: 23199371.

13. Angela R. Kamer and others, "Periodontal Inflammation in Relation to Cognitive Function in an Older Danish Adult Population," *Journal of Alzheimer's Disease* 28, no. 3 (2012): 613–624, DOI: 10.3233/JAD-2011-102004, PMID: 22045483.

14. Ide M, Harris M, Stevens A, Sussams R, Hopkins V, Culliford D, et al. (2016) Periodontitis and Cognitive Decline in Alzheimer's Disease. PLoS ONE 11(3): e0151081. doi:10.1371/journal.pone.0151081

15. Mutter J, Curth A, Naumann J, Deth R, Walach H. Does inorganic mercury play a role in Alzheimer's disease? A systematic review and an integrated molecular mechanism. J Alzheimers Dis. 2010;22(2):357-74. PMID 20847438

16. Mutter J, Naumann J, Schneider R, Walach H. Mercury and Alzheimer's disease. Fortschr Neurol Psychiatr. 2007 Sep;75(9):528-38. Epub 2007 Jul 12. PMID 17628833.

17. Houston MC. Role of Mercury Toxicity in Hypertension, Cardiovascular Disease, and StrokeJ Clin Hypertens (Greenwich) 2011 Aug;13(8):621-7. PMID 21806773.

18. Frustaci A, Magnavita N, Chimenti C, Caldarulo M, Sabbioni E, Pietra R, Cellini C, Possati GF, Maseri A. J Am Coll Cardiol. 1999 May; 33(6):1578-83. PMID 10334427.

19. Siblerud RL. The relationship between mercury from dental amalgam and the cardiovascular system. Sci Total Environ. 1990 Dec 1; 99(1-2):23-35. PMID 2270468.

20. Boyd Haley, PhD, Amalgams and Alzheimer's Disease: https://dentalwellness4u.com/mercury/ref1. html#A17alzheimers

21. Dr. Tom McGuire's DentalWellness4u.com.

22. American Dental Association Council on Scientific Affairs, Dental Mercury Hygiene Recommendations: The Journal of the American Dental Association, Vol. 134, Issue 11, p1498–1499.

23. Mutter J, Naumann J, Schneider R, Walach H. Mercury and Alzheimer's disease. Fortschr Neurol Psychiatr. 2007 Sep;75(9):528-38. Epub 2007 Jul 12. PMID: 17628833.

24. Pendergrass JC, Haley BE, Vimy MJ, Winfield SA, Lorscheider FL. Mercury vapor inhalation inhibits binding of GTP to tubulin in rat brain: similarity to a molecular lesion in Alzheimer diseased brain. Neurotoxicology. 1997; 18(2):315-24. PMID 9291481.

25. Division of Sleep Medicine at Harvard Medical School, Sleep and Disease Risk: http://healthysleep.med.harvard.edu/healthy/matters/consequences/sleep-and-disease-risk

26. Centers for Disease Control and Prevention, Mental Health, Depression: http://www.cdc.gov/mentalhealth/basics/mental-illness/depression.htm

27. American Psychiatric Association. Quick Reference to the Diagnostic Criteria from DSM-IV. Washington, DC. American Psychiatric Press, Inc. 1994.

28. Coulombe JA, Reid GJ, Boyle MH, Racine Y. Sleep problems, tiredness, and psychological symptoms among healthy adolescents. J Pediatr Psychol 2010; [Epub ahead of print].

29. Moreh E, Jacobs JM, Stessman J. Fatigue, function, and mortality in older adults. J Gerontol A Biol Sci Med Sci 2010 [Epub ahead of print].

30. Itzhaki RF, Wozniak MA. Herpes simplex virus type 1 in Alzheimer's disease: the enemy within. J Alzheimers Dis. 2008 May;13(4):393-405. PMID: 18487848.

31. Letenneur L, et al. Seropositivity to herpes simplex virus antibodies and risk of Alzheimer's disease: a population-based cohort study. PLoS One. 2008; 3(11):e3637. PMID: 18982063.

32. Raji CA, et al. Longitudinal Relationships between Caloric Expenditure and Gray Matter in the Cardiovascular Health Study, Journal of Alzheimer's Disease (http://content. iospress.com/journals/journal-of-alzheimers-disease), vol. Preprint, no. Preprint, pp. 1-11, 2016 , Published 11 March 2016. DOI: 10.3233/JAD-160057

33. Dr. David Perlmutter, Drug Free Approach Cuts Alzheimer's Risk In Half, posted May 6, 2016, on GreenMedInfo.com

Ch. 17 Chair Side Investigations: Finding the Missing Link to Restart and Renew Your Health

1. Jäkel, Anne; Von Hauenschild, Philip (2012). "A systematic review to evaluate the clinical benefits of craniosacral therapy". *Complementary Therapies in Medicine*. **20** (6): 456–65. PMID 23131379. doi:10.1016/j.ctim.2012.07.009.

2. Discover CranioSacral Therapy: The Health Power of Gentle Touch. Upledger Institute International, 2016.

3. William Garner Sutherland, D.O., Teaching in the Science of Osteopathy. Sutherland Cranial Teaching Foundation, Inc. Fort Worth, TX 1990.

4. Harold Ives Magoun, D.O., Osteopathy in the Cranial Field: The Application to the Cranium of the Principles of Osteopathy, Based on the Arduous Study and Keen Clinical Observation of William Garner Sutherland. utherland Cranial Teaching Foundation, Inc. Fort Worth, TX 1996.

5. Torseten Liem, Cranial Osteopathy: A Practical Textbook. Eastland Press, Seattle, WA 2009

6. Ernest @. Retzlaff, Frederic L. Mitchell, Je. (Eds), The Cranium and Its Sutures. Springer-Verlag Berlin Heidelberg 1987.

7. John E. Upledger, D.O., Jon D. Vredevoodg, MFA, Craniosacral Therapy. Eastland Press, Seattle, WA 1983.

8. John E. Upledger, D.O., Your Inner Physician and You: CranioSacral therapy and SomatoEmotional Release. North Atlantic Books, Berkeley, CA 1997.

9. Upledger.com: Discover CranioSacral Therapy: http://www.upledger.com/therapies/index.php.

Ch. 18 Your Child's Dental-facial Development: Nutritional Lessons From Pottenger's Cats

1. Francis M. Pottenger Jr., MD. Pottenger's Cats: A Study in Nutrition, 2nd ed. (Lemon Grove, CA: Price-Pottenger Nutrition Foundation, 1995.

2. Francis M. Pottenger Jr., MD. Pottenger's Cats: A Study in Nutrition, 2nd ed., p. 22. (Lemon Grove, CA: Price-Pottenger Nutrition Foundation, 1995.

3. Francis M. Pottenger Jr., MD. *Pottenger's Cats: A Study in Nutrition,* 2nd ed., p. 41.Weston A. Price, *Nutrition and Physical Degeneration* (Lemon Grove, CA: Price-Pottenger Nutrition Foundation, 2008). An earlier version of the book can be read at http://gutenberg.net.au/ebooks02/0200251h.html or http://journeytoforever.org/farm_library/price/pricetoc.html.

4. Francis M. Pottenger Jr., MD. *Pottenger's Cats: A Study in Nutrition,* 2nd ed., p. 42. (Lemon Grove, CA: Price-Pottenger Nutrition Foundation, 1995.(Lemon Grove, CA: Price-Pottenger Nutrition Foundation, 1995.

5. Francis M. Pottenger Jr., MD. *Pottenger's Cats: A Study in Nutrition,* 2nd ed., p.15. (Lemon Grove, CA: Price-Pottenger Nutrition Foundation, 1995.

Made in United States
Orlando, FL
04 March 2023

30680362R00185